Aging at Home: How the Elderly Adjust Their Housing Without Moving

ABOUT THE AUTHORS

Raymond J. Struyk, PhD, is Director of the Center for International Activities at The Urban Institute in Washington, D.C. and Senior Research Associate at the Center for Public Finance. As a senior analyst in the fields of housing and community development, he has extensive experience in policy formulation and analysis. His numerous publications reflect his interest in many aspects of the housing situation of the poor and the elderly. He is currently engaged in several projects exploring the relationship between housing circumstances of the elderly and the likelihood of institutional placement. Dr. Struyk is an associate editor of the *Journal of Housing for the Elderly*.

Harold M. Katsura, MCRP, is Research Associate II at The Urban Institute in Washington, D.C. Since joining the Institute in 1984, he has been involved with a wide variety of international and domestic projects. In the domestic area, he has worked primarily on evaluations of federal programs, studies of the housing situation of the elderly, and analysis of proposed housing policies. Mr. Katsura received his Masters degree in City and Regional Planning from Harvard University's John F. Kennedy School of Government where he specialized in housing and community development.

Aging at Home: How the Elderly Adjust Their Housing Without Moving

Raymond J. Struyk
Harold M. Katsura

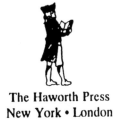

The Haworth Press
New York • London

Aging at Home: How the Elderly Adjust Their Housing Without Moving has also been published as *Journal of Housing for the Elderly*, Volume 4, Number 2, Fall/Winter 1987.

The Haworth Press, Inc., 10 Alice Street, Binghamton, NY 13904-1580 USA

Library of Congress Cataloging-in-Publication Data

Struyk, Raymond J.
   Aging at home.

   "Published as Journal of Housing for the elderly, volume 4, number 2, fall/winter 1987" — Verso t.p.
   Bibliography: p.
   1. Aged — Housing — United States. 2. Aged — United States — Dwellings. 3. Dwellings — United States-Remodeling. I. Katsura, Harold M. II. Title.
HD7287.92.U5S87 1988   363.5'9   88-2738
ISBN 0-86656-736-4

Aging at Home: How the Elderly Adjust Their Housing Without Moving

CONTENTS

Acknowledgements

A number of individuals and organizations contributed importantly to the completion of the work reported in this volume. Stephen Gayle and others at the University of Pennsylvania who were working on the Community Development Strategies Evaluation for the U.S. Department of Housing and Urban Development generously shared with us the rich data set they had developed. The National Opinion Research Center of the University of Chicago carried out the extensive survey work done as part of this project efficiently and professionally. The attrition rates in our panel sample were very low, a tribute to the solid performance of the group of interviewers who conducted the total of seven interviews. We also want to thank James Zais for his help in the initial stages of the project and Sandra Newman for reviewing our work at various stages.

Finally, we gratefully acknowledge the support for this work provided by the National Institute of Aging, U.S. Department of Health and Human Services, under Grant No. 5R01AG03145.

Chapter 1

Introduction and Summary

The sharp increase in the number of elderly in the United States – and their share of the total population – in the years ahead is widely recognized. Between 1980 and 2020, they will double from 26 to 52 million persons, or from 27 to 30% of the population. Moreover, the share of elderly over age 75 will surge from 40% in 1980 to 50% in 2000 and then decline somewhat by 2020 only to resurge again (Table 1.1).

These trends have profound implications for the housing requirements of Americans. A steady increase of those living alone is certainly expected, as is some increase in the share of elderly who choose to take in roomers or boarders for economic reasons or for the help a boarder could provide. As the number of persons over age 75 mounts, the need for specially modified dwellings and additional support services will rise as well. In the past the great majority of help of this type was provided by family members; but with reduced kinship networks becoming a fact because of smaller family sizes, a larger share of such caring will have to be formally provided – a good deal of it in institutions unless there are changes in federal policies to make it easier for the elderly to obtain such services while remaining in the community. Indeed, without such changes the cost of federal health care financing programs will be 5.4% of GNP in the year 2020, compared with 2.3% in 1980 (Palmer & Torrey, 1984, Table 1).

Raymond J. Struyk is Senior Research Associate and Harold M. Katsura is Research Associate for The Urban Institute, 2100 M Street, NW, Washington, DC 20037.

1

TABLE 1.1

THE ABSOLUTE AND RELATIVE SIZES
OF AGED POPULATION

	No. of Aged (in mill.) (1)	% Increase in the No. of Aged Over Past Decade (2)	Aged as a % of Population (3)	As a Percentage of Total Aged Persons Aged 65-75 (4)	75+ (5)
1960	17.1	34.7	9.1	65.5	34.5
1970	20.7	20.6	9.7	60.6	39.4
1980	26.3	27.3	11.1	59.9	40.1
1990	32.7	24.1	12.6	56.7	43.3
2000	36.3	11.3	13.1	50.3	49.7
2010	40.7	12.0	13.9	51.7	48.3
2020	53.2	30.8	17.3	58.0	42.0
2030	66.2	24.4	20.8	52.9	47.1
2040	69.0	4.2	21.2	43.8	56.2

Source: Palmer and Torrey (1984), Table 2, p. 126.

Note: The aged include the total population eligible for Social
Security and Medicare benefits who are sixty-five years old or
older. Historically this number has been about 800,000 higher
than the Census count of the United States aged population (age
sixty-five and over) because it includes people who live
overseas.

The housing arrangements of the elderly are an important element in designing cost-effective interventions to help them remain in the community. Its importance derives from the fact that cost of housing services constitutes a large fraction of the total expenses of living in the community—or in an institution. The quality of the home environment is, of course, a key determinant to a person's quality of life, particularly among the elderly who spend a larger share of time at home. Finally, housing can effect whether an elderly person remains in the community in several direct ways. First, housing conditions can have a dramatic effect on a chronically ill or disabled person's ability to function in performing everyday activities (Thomas, 1983). For example, installing a bathroom on the first floor of a two-story home could determine whether a person with severe mobility problems could remain in his home. Second, certain housing characteristics have been found to be correlated with a family's willingness to care for an elderly relative (Sussman, 1979). Third, the attributes of the unit can effect the ability of care providers from outside of the household to render services. Presence of complete kitchen and bathroom facilities, for example, may be essential (Newman, 1985). In short, housing circumstances may matter a great deal in determining who is able to remain in the community. Moreover, it is essential to recognize that the housing situation will have to be adjusted over time as household composition and housing needs change.

Among the critical background information for designing appropriate incentives for and assistance with timely adjustments in housing circumstances that will help the elderly remain in the community is understanding the reasons households now make such adjustments. Additionally, knowing these behavioral relationships will shed light on other decisions the elderly make about their living environment and living arrangements.

The particular focus of the analysis presented here is adjustments to the housing "bundle" made without relocating, i.e., the in-place housing adjustments of the elderly. The present state of knowledge about such adjustments is extremely limited. We are virtually wholly ignorant about the incidence of such adjustments as changing the use of rooms or making modifications to the dwelling (like installing the bathroom cited above) in response to mobility limitations by a household member. Obviously, we know even less about what factors cause such adjustments — and which act as intervening variables to make such adjustments unnecessary. For example, the presence of personal services from family members may sharply reduce the need for changes to the dwelling. Certainly, we have no idea about the probable delay between the time of a major change, such as the loss of income that may come with the death of a spouse or the onset of activity limitations, and the corresponding adjustment to the dwelling unit.

The purpose of this monograph is to report the findings of a research project designed to fill the void in the existing knowledge about the incidence of in-place adjustments and the factors causing them. As suggested earlier, in-place adjustments along with shifting to a different dwelling are the two ways a household has of altering the bundle of housing services it consumes. Typically, one thinks of larger changes being effected by relocating. But the exceptions are certainly numerous. One can think, for example, of people making major additions or alterations to their home rather than moving—a phenomenon more common in recent years as the cost for home-owners of switching homes has increased because of the higher mortgage interest rate on the new unit.

Four separate types of housing adjustments are analyzed here: changes in the use of rooms; modifications to the dwelling to facili-tate its use by persons with physical impairments; taking in roomers or boarders; and, adjusting the amount of repairs and improvements to the unit which are undertaken. As far as we know, this is the first time such a comprehensive set of adjustments has been studied for the same sample of households.

The literature on the determinants of residential mobility empha-sizes the idea that the household relocates when the present housing bundle diverges sufficiently from the bundle currently desired that the benefits from moving will more than compensate for the associ-ated costs. In short, when the "housing disequilibrium" becomes great enough, the family shifts to a different unit. Factors producing this disequilibrium are such things as changes in economic position, household size and composition, and the ability of household mem-bers to use the unit (or stated conversely, the onset of activity limi-tations by some members of the household). The same general logic applies to in-place adjustments. However, because the cost of many in-place adjustments is quite modest, one expects to observe a suc-cession of such adjustments with the adaption of the unit toward the desired bundle evolving over time, albeit by fits and starts.

Our objective is to examine the frequency of change in those factors that may be causing housing adjustments to take place, to identify those with the more prominent causal effects on adjust-ments, and to examine the frequency of in-place adjustments. A major simplification in the analysis is that we examine a sample containing only homeowners who live in single-family dwellings (as opposed to two- or four-plexes or multiunit condominiums). Still, almost 70% of elderly headed households live in such units.

STUDY SAMPLE AND DATA COLLECTION

As intriguing and important as the issues raised above are, they have been very little studied, mostly because of the absence of necessary time-series data. As part of this project, an appropriate data set was assembled which contains almost five years of information on 364 households as of the end of the observation period in the fall of 1984. This project extended an ongoing panel survey of households, a sample drawn from selected neighborhoods in seven large cities. Consequently, the resulting sample of households used in this analysis cannot be considered to be strictly representative of the elderly living in the urban areas.

The analysis sample contains 187 households headed by a non-elderly person and 177 households headed by an elderly person (someone 60 years of age or older at about the one-third point of the observation period). Samples for both groups were included to permit us to isolate those types of changes in housing and other factors that are special to the elderly.

This study fielded the last three of a total of five waves of household surveys, each wave interviewing the same household. (Relocating households were not followed.) Because the purpose of the study for which the sample was originally drawn was different from ours, considerable modification to the survey instrument was made between the second and third survey waves. Nevertheless, substantial continuity was maintained between the contents and specific questions in the two instruments. In addition to the household surveys, there was also an inspection of the dwellings and a "windshield survey" of neighborhoods at the start of the survey period. The final data set contains information in the following areas for each household for periods of three to five years: housing adjustments; dwelling quality and configuration; economic position including income, assets, and housing expenses; household composition and living arrangements; extent of social interaction through church attendance, "club" meetings and contact with children living outside of the home; limitations in performing a variety of daily activities; informal and formal supporting services received; and intentions about relocating.

HIGHLIGHTS

The results of this project fall into three distinct groups. The first is simply the documentation of the amount of in-place housing adjustments ongoing; how much change is occurring on an annual basis? The second concerns how these adjustment unfold over time and the extent of change in those factors — economic, health, demographic, social support — that we believe determine the presence or absence of housing adjustments. The final group of results is for the statistical modeling of the determinants of each of the housing adjustments being studied.

The Extent of In-Place Housing Adjustments

The incidence of the various housing adjustments is summarized in Table 1.2 separately for households headed by an elderly person and those headed by a nonelderly person. The rates are for the last two years of the approximately five year observation period. Only a very small percentage of households had a roomer or boarder present or changed the use of rooms within their homes over this period. A rather surprisingly high 10% of elderly headed and 5% of the nonelderly headed households undertook modifications to their homes to facilitate their use by a physically impaired family member. Taken together, these figures indicate that about 8% of elderly headed and 6% of nonelderly headed households make one of these three types of housing adjustment *each year*. These rates can be put into perspective by noting that about 3.3% of the elderly and 13% of the nonelderly homeowners adjust their housing circumstances by changing residence each year.[1] Hence, rates of in-place adjustments for the elderly are at least double those achieved by relocating.

Repairs and improvements are associated with the types of adjustments just reviewed and with longer term strategies of housing upkeep and investment. A central hypothesis considered here is that there is a cohort of elderly homeowners who, because of economic or health circumstances, decides implicitly to draw down on the equity in their homes through a program of undermaintenance. Similarly, we are interested in which households persistently are investing in their homes. The last two rows of figures in Table 1.2 show

TABLE 1.2

INCIDENCE OF HOUSING ADJUSTMENTS BY
AGE OF HOUSEHOLD HEAD
(percents)

	Elderly-headed households	Non-elderly headed households
Roomer or boarder present, in last 2 years	3	1
At least one room use change in last 2 years	5	6
Dwelling modified to assist impaired person, last 2 years	10	5
Dwelling repairs and improvements over last 2 years:		
o made repairs in both years	69	80
o made moderate sized repair in at least one year[a]	77	83
o made major repair in at least one year[b]	19	22
o only small or no repairs in both years	20	14
o no repairs	5	3

a. Moderate repairs are those costing between $100 and $1000, inclusive.

b. Major repairs or improvements are those costing over $1,000.

that 20% of the elderly in our sample undertook little or no repair activity over two years and that they were somewhat more likely to this than their nonelderly counterparts; however, the differences between the two groups are not large. Similarly, the elderly as a group are undertaking repair and improvements—even large improvements to their homes—at quite high rates. Still, they undertake fewer such repairs and investments and each year they spend less than their more youthful counterparts. The overall pattern is one in which properties are indeed largely being maintained, and disinvesting households are a definite minority and comparable in size with the nonelderly.

A final point concerns the extent to which multiple types of adjustments are being made by the same households. Even when we examine the adjustments made over the full five year period, we find little evidence of households making more than one type of housing change. The only exception to this is between those making major improvements to their homes and those modifying their homes to facilitate its use by an impaired member where a clear pattern of overlap is evident.

Dynamics of the Process

As suggested earlier, prior to this analysis we had very little idea about the pattern of change over the years in the way the elderly used and maintained their homes and in the factors that could directly effect housing adjustments. How stable are living arrangements? How dynamic are the incomes of the elderly compared to the nonelderly? Among those elderly who do not relocate, are their problems with doing various daily activities better thought of as episodic or chronic?

Three types of housing adjustments—bringing a roomer or boarder into the home, changing the use of the room, and modifying the dwelling so as to better meet the needs of an impaired person—all occur on a highly discrete basis and households rarely undertake them. There is a low average incidence and typically a household will only make one such change over a several year period.

A similar pattern of discrete undertakings also applies to a considerable range of dwelling repair and improvement activity. While most households do make some repairs or improvements each year, the type of actions, their cost, and their number vary sharply for the same household year by year. The degree of discontinuity is greater for elderly households than their more youthful counterparts. Few households were found to neglect repair and improvements year after year.

Regarding the dwellings occupied, these homes were found to exhibit an impressive amount of structural problems (as rated by trained inspectors) at the start of the observation period. But if the evidence on persistency of various dwelling problems which we were able to track over the period is any guide, most of these problems are remedied once they are discovered by their owner-occupants. Very few units show a pattern of problems remaining unattended over several years.

The layout of the units included in the sample is surprisingly adaptable to families with members with activity limitations. Most have their living space on a single floor. And only about 20% do not have both a bedroom and bath on the first floor. These unit attributes sharply reduce the need for extensive dwelling modifications.

The overall picture of the older households included in this study is definitely one of evident aging over the observation period, as indicated by reduced working, the increase in the number of single person households to 35% of the total by the end of the period, and the decline in the share of households that are simple husband-wife households. In addition, all of the information points to there being a great deal of churning in living arrangements and in the number of persons present in a household from year to year. This dynamic pattern suggests that there may be considerable opportunity for living arrangements to be modified to provide supportive services without the elderly household having to relocate.

The elderly are seen to have a wide-range of contacts outside of the home which presumably stimulate them and which can be a source of assistance when needed, particularly on an episodic basis. Among various sources those through the church and those with their children are clearly paramount, to judge by regularity and frequency of contact. Importantly, the frequency of contact with children was found to be highly stable over time, despite a good deal of residential mobility on the part of the children. We hypothesize that contact with children may be important for making housing adjustments, both for directly accomplishing them and for providing advice and support. Those lacking such aid may well make fewer adjustments of the type being studied here.

The picture of activity limitations and corresponding supportive services received is very definitely one of episodic problems and responses. While both activity limitations and assistance are highly prevalent each year, there is little incidence of either persisting over a several year period. Apparently those with more serious and persistent problems are unable to remain in their homes.

The information on the economic circumstances of households points to a combination of stability over time for most households and considerable change in the economic ranking of others over the observation period. Such income or wealth changes, especially reductions, could strongly effect the timing of undertaking major dwelling modifications or improvements; or it could cause the family to consider taking in a roomer or boarder.

Multivariate Analyses

In the final part of this work we employ multivariate techniques with the goal of identifying the broad relationships present between each of the housing adjustments and the factors we have hypothesized to causally effect the occurrence of such adjustments. The ability to successfully carry out these analyses was somewhat limited by the small sample sizes involved and the small number of some adjustments that were observed over the five-year period. Nevertheless, some distinct patterns did emerge from the analysis. Because the patterns for the elderly differ from those for the nonelderly, we concentrate in this summary on the findings for households headed by an elderly person.

Changes in the *use of rooms* within a dwelling are systematically driven by the activity limitations of the household members. While severe limitations on the part of a spouse have especially powerful effects, limitations experienced by the respondent and the presence in the household of someone else with physical impairments also significantly increase the likelihood of room use changes. On the other hand, the receipt of help by the spouse from outside of the home is a strong offsetting factor. Interestingly, receipt of meal services for an extended period or the start of receipt of transportation services provided by an agency are positively associated with room usage changes — possibly indicating shifts made to make using these other services more convenient. Men living alone are over 10% more likely to make such room use changes than other types of households. Finally, economic circumstances do not appear to play an important role in determining whether housing adjustments of this type are undertaken.

The multivariate models estimated to explain the probability that a household would *take in a roomer or boarder* over the period yielded quite weak results, indicating the lack of systematic association between this type of housing adjustment and the factors hypothesized here to be causal agents. Still, some worthwhile findings were obtained. If the respondent had experienced severe mobility limitations and had been receiving some help from outside the home for an extended period, the likelihood of having borders in the home is sharply higher than for others. Changes in these statuses over the period reduce this likelihood, presumably such changes prevent other households in this situation from executing possible plans to take in a roomer. Multiperson households and men living alone appear to be more willing to take a boarder than elderly women living alone, after controlling for other factors. This finding is consistent with women being concerned about having strangers in their homes. There is also some indication that incomes falling over the period — not low initial incomes — may be a factor pushing households to accept boarders.

The likelihood that an elderly household will *modify its dwelling so as to be more useful to a physically impaired household member* is also determined significantly by the presence of members with activity limitations. Again, such limitations on the part of the spouse are especially important. Both activity limitations per se and the use by the spouse of special equipment to assist with mobility (e.g., walker, wheelchair) are strongly correlated with this type of adjustment. Counterbalancing the limitations to some degree are the receipt of services and the presence of social support outside of the home: starting to see at least one child once or more each week, having meals brought to the home over an extended period, and regularly attending a senior center all lower the probability that a modification will be made.

Economic position does not play much of a role in determining the likelihood of this type of housing adjustment occurring, suggesting that one way or another those households who badly needed to make dwelling modifications get them done. Additionally, it is of interest to note that changes in the economic position of households over the full observation period were consistently not significant determinants of such changes. Additionally, for the elderly the configuration of multistory homes did not effect the likelihood of an adjustment being made, although for the nonelderly the presence of both a bedroom and a bathroom on the first floor of such a unit reduces the likelihood of a modification by about 7%.

As suggested earlier, the *analysis of repairs and improvements* differs qualitatively from the other housing adjustments under consideration because they are not readily identifiable one-time events. Rather, households may change their level of activity and maintain it over a period of years, with the effects of such shifts only gradually becoming evident. The findings in this area can be illustrated for the probability of a household undertaking some repair or improvement activity in both of the final years of the observation period and the probability that in both years, given that it undertook repairs, the household spent more than the median amount expended for repairs among sample households making some repairs.

The economic position of the household is clearly more important for repairs and improvements than for the other adjustments. Especially with regard to the likelihood of spending more than the median amount, income level at the start of the two year period over which the repair activity of the dependent variable is defined was important. Households in the lowest income quartile are about 25% less likely to spend more than the median amount in successive years than a household in the highest income quartile. Dwelling conditions play less of a causal role than we have anticipated. Substantial dwelling defects present at the baseline (year one) turn out to be a good predictor of the *lack* of future repair activity in the final two years. The presence of problems with leaking basements, heating systems and the like — measured each year during the period — were found to exert little measurable influence on repair activity. On the other hand, the stated intention to move prior to the two years over which the dependent variable is measured is consistently associated with considerably higher levels of repairs and improvements. Apparently, plans to move lead to more vigilance in maintaining the unit, even if no move occurs for a couple of years.

In general, activity limitations and receipt of social support and assistance from outside of the home are less important in explaining repairs than they are for other housing adjustments. But some of these effects are captured by the household undertaking a dwelling modification which does significantly raise the probability of a sustained high level of repair activity. Living arrangements (and implied levels of potential support within the home) have only limited influence on repair activity.

There are a few direct implications for public policy that can be drawn from these findings. One of these concerns programs designed to encourage the elderly to repair and improve their homes, perhaps as part of broader neighborhood preservation strategies. The findings show income — or economic resources, more broadly — to be definitely important. And, indeed, the provision of cash grants to low income elderly homeowners in the Experimental Housing Allowance Program resulted in a sharp rise in expenditure levels for maintenance and repairs. But the results also show that the best predictor of low levels of repair activity among the elderly is the presence of significant problems three years before the start of the period over which we studied repair activity. To reach these households — who would be unlikely to be able to bring their homes up to the standards needed to qualify for a housing allowance payment — would require a very different approach, presumably one characterized by intensive outreach activities.[2]

The second area for which these findings may have direct bearing concerns the "home matching" programs which are being spawned around the country at a very high rate. Such programs typically aim to match someone looking for a low-rent room with elderly homeowners who live in units that contain more space than they need. The prototypical homeowner is conceived to be a woman living alone. Our results suggest that this phenomenon is still quite rare. Moreover, consistent with other studies, we find that matches are of short duration: no one in our sample maintained a boarder (or series of boarders) over the entire observation period. Such churning means that the administrative cost associated with a full year of a shared unit could be quite high, as it would involve multiple matches. Finally, our findings point to elderly women living alone being *less* likely to accept such arrangements, at least as the arrangements have been presented in the past.

The final observation concerns possible public policies that might be designed to promote appropriate room use changes and dwelling modifications where they are needed to make the home better match the needs of a physically impaired person. The short message is that such interventions must be approached very cautiously. Our findings suggest that households have worked out careful arrangements to meet their needs that involve a wide variety of sources. The key to successful public intervention will be for changes to the dwelling of this type to complement ongoing assistance. This in turn means that mass, formula-driven programs will probably not work; rather a more tailored approach, involving greater front-end administrative effort is necessary.

NOTES

1. Schneider, Stahl, & Struyk (1985), Table 2.4; tabulation of figures from the Annual Housing Survey for 1978.
2. For more on such programs, see Struyk (1985).

Chapter 2

Conceptual Framework

In this chapter we outline the model that underlies all of the analysis presented in subsequent chapters. The decision to undertake adjustments in the use and configuration of the dwelling is presented in the conventional demand and supply framework favored by economists. For ease of presentation, we begin with a static model; later, greater realism is added with a more complete dynamic formulation. At the outset only a single type of adjustment — making "repairs" to the home — is considered.

The presentation of the basic model in the first section of the chapter is fairly brief and compressed, spending little time discussing the role of individual causal factors and types of housing adjustments. We remedy these deficiencies in the remaining sections. In one we discuss the various types of housing adjustments, and in the other we elaborate on the role of the causal factors, based in part on the findings of a host of prior studies. As part of the latter, there is an overview of the expected relationship among various causal factors and different types of in-place housing adjustments.

It may be worth stressing that the purpose of this discussion is to provide a context within which to conduct the empirical analysis. It does not purport to represent a new theoretical model for discussing this problem, although the discussion may be more complete than prior ones.[1]

CONCEPTUAL MODEL

Static Formulation

The demand for repairs or repair activities, D, can be thought of as derived from the demand for housing services. Therefore, the determinants of D closely parallel those for housing services. These can be summarized as:

$$D = D (Y,A,r,HH,SS,H/I,C,N,SI,D_{t-1},P_1,P_2,P_3,P_4. \quad (1)$$

Y is the household's current income and A are assets. Assets are especially important because: (1) they can be directly used to finance repairs; (2) they influence the household's judgment as to the fraction of income it feels it can devote to housing; and (3) they are indicative of the household's permanent income. The households' discount rate, r, can have a strong negative influence on D, as the household becomes increasingly aged, i.e., the household anticipates obtaining little enjoyment out of investments made in the unit. On the other hand, this may be offset by a strong bequest factor, so that r may have little effect on demand (Blinder, 1976).

Household composition or living arrangements, HH, influence D largely through the demand of individual members for a certain quantity of housing services, all things being equal (e.g., one spouse may be more sensitive to dwelling conditions than another). SS is the extent of support services provided by those not living in the household, ranging from family members to agencies. Those providing such services may make the resident aware of previously unobserved or discounted problems with his or her dwelling. The service provider may also help make arrangements for having the repair made. Health problems and physical impairments (H/I) may affect the demand for repairs and maintenance by making the installation of grab bars and similar items a necessity.

The condition of the dwelling, C, is an obvious determinant; in the extreme, repairs would have to be undertaken for the dwelling to remain habitable. N is the condition of the neighborhood; if it is declining, the return to maintenance activity would be sharply reduced, since property values in the area would be low to begin with. N also includes the extent and type of public investment recently made in the neighborhood—improving street lighting, curbs and gutters, recreational facilities—which may also affect the return on investment. Finally, SI is the amount of social interaction between the household members and others in their neighborhood; the hypothesis here is that greater contact with others will make the household more sensitive to the condition of the dwelling, and thus influence the extent of upkeep. In addition, more contact may well generate further sources of assistance in getting some types of repairs made. The demand for repairs in previous periods, D_{t-1}, is included to reflect what economists term "habit formation" effects on consumption. In this case households have become accustomed to a certain degree of upkeep and unit quality, and this will effect future consumption decisions. This effect is likely to be especially significant for older households, and one expects such habit formation to have an impact on repair activity quite independent of unit conditions, at least to the degree we can measure them.

Four price terms are included in the demand function, one for each of the relevant types of suppliers; P_1 is the price per unit of repairs if the household is making the repair itself; P_2 is the price if a friend or relative is making the repair; P_3 is the price of employing someone else to make the repair; and P_4 is the price when assistance is provided by government or other service providers. As outlined below, each source of supply involves a different production technology and possibly different factor prices. The household chooses among the different suppliers of repairs on the basis of price.

The formulation presented thus far tacitly assumes a "repair" to be a homogeneous good, regardless of who supplies it. It is quite conceivable, however, that repairs are perceived to be differentiated goods depending on who supplies them. It is arguable that a job one does himself or herself is viewed as a superior good, since one knows "the job was done right." In recognition of the possible differentiation, "repairs" (and the demand for them) can be distinguished by their source of supply — D_1, D_2, D_3 — in much the same way consumers distinguished among automobiles or cereals.[2]

If repairs are differentiated goods, in demand as well as supply, the demand function for D (eq. 1) would be replaced by a group of functions, one for each D_i type of repairs, distinguished by the main source of labor. One can easily write a reduced-form equation for each D_i as follows:

$$D_i = D_i (Y,A,r,HH,SS,H/I,C,N,SI,D_{t-1},P_i,P_j,P_k,D_j,D_k \ldots) \ i \neq j \quad (2)$$

The levels of D_i are clearly determined jointly, since the P_j and hence the relative attractiveness of the jth type of repair depends on how much of the jth activity has been demanded in the relevant time period.[3] This is true except for contractors whose supply schedule to the individual household is flat — that is, contractors supplying as much as demanded at a constant price. In other words, if self-made repairs are the most preferred, the demand for the contractor repairs would depend on the relative price of self-repairs. The price would rise sharply as the household members make more repairs them- selves, reflecting greater opportunity cost of devoting more time to such activity.[4] Assuming the demand for a repair activity — fixing a broken window, for example — the choice among the differentiated goods depends on the household's taste, other demand determi- nants, and the relative prices of the supply sources, which in turn are driven by the total demand for each repair type to date in the relevant time period.

This line of reasoning suggests that a mix of repair types ob- served over an extended time period would be sensitive to the time interval between individual repairs. If repairs were clustered, one would predict a higher fraction of contractor repairs; less bunching would imply a lower implicit wage rate of the household and/or relative.[5] Thus, the timing of repairs (or other in-place adjustments) is critically important to the analysis.

Four types of suppliers are distinguished in Figure 2.1, which depicts a supply function for each type. In the four graphs, P is the price per unit for repair services and Q is the quantity of the services provided in a specific time period. Panel (a) illustrates the provision of services by the household itself. The "price" here is an implicit one — the cost perceived by the household of doing various tasks for itself.[6] The supply schedule shows an upward slope. This is because the tasks become increasingly more difficult for members of the elderly household as more is done, because of their lack of stamina and possible physical impairments. The difference in the actual placement of the supply schedules with three levels of impairment (H/I) is suggested in the figure; the greater the level of impairment the more costly it is for the household to provide any quality of services. Similar shifts in the schedules could be caused by the pres- ence of children or a spouse to help with various chores.

Panel (b) of Figure 2.1 depicts the provision of services by friends or family members not living in the household. Again, the schedule is upward-sloping, this time because of the hypothesized

FIGURE 2.1

Alternative Suppliers of Repair Services

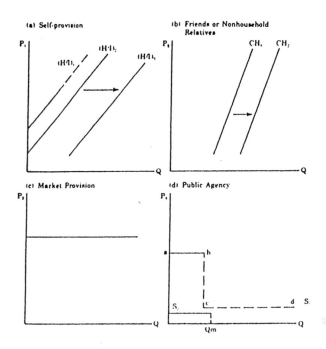

(a) Self-provision   (b) Friends or Nonhousehold Relatives   (c) Market Provision   (d) Public Agency

aversion of these informal suppliers to providing services as the amount increases. Presumably, this aversion begins after some level of services has been reached, although this discontinuity is not shown in the figure. The steepness of the schedule is based on the observation that the elderly homeowners seem to avoid asking friends or relatives for help in making repairs to their dwelling (Struyk-Soldo, Chap. 4). Finally, note that the schedule is shown to shift out with more friends or relatives (NH) residing within a short commuting distance.

Since the demand for repairs by any individual household is slight comparing to the total services available from commercial vendors, the elderly household is shown in Panel (c) as being able to purchase all desired services at the market place, M_1. However, this price excludes the cost to the household of acquiring such services. For some, the effort required to find and negotiate with a contractor is substantial and for them the price per unit rises to M_2 or M_3.

Public provision of services can be supplied under a variety of arrangements, two of which are illustrated in Panel (d). Note that this figure applies only to those households meeting the program requirements. The first schedule (S_1) is a program under which the household pays some price for the initial set of services in the year (line segment ab) and a negligible amount thereafter for as many services as it needs (cd). By contrast, S_2 is a program under which the only cost to the household is its time, but a fixed maximum amount of services (Q_m) is available to it.

In light of the foregoing, the supply function for the household providing repair services itself can be written as:

$$P_1 = P_1(M, HH, H/I, SS). \quad (3)$$

M is the price per unit of nonlabor inputs and HH is the household type. The concept is, for example, that husband-wife couples, working together, may be able to perform many domestic duties at a more reasonable level of exertion than an individual living alone. The presence of children in the home is included in the definition of household composition on the same grounds. Health/physical impairments (H/I), of course, reflect the greater difficulty of those in poorer health doing various domestic tasks. On the other hand, receipt of services (SS) can have a countervailing impact. A person providing assistance can effect the "supply of maintenance services" to the dwelling in several distinct ways. First, the helper might be directly involved in accomplishing repairs. For example, the assistance might be chore services, under which particular jobs might include holding a ladder or helping patch a crack in wall plaster preparatory to painting. A second effect is simply a direct substitution of labor: the elderly are able to expend their limited energy on maintenance, if other work is done for them. Finally, the assistance might be in arranging for work to be done either privately or by a public agency.

The function for friends and nonresident family members is the following:

$$P_2 = P_2(M,NH,Z) \quad (4)$$

M is the price per unit of nonlabor inputs. NH is the number of friends and nonresident family members in the area, and Z is the actual proximity of such individuals to the elderly household. The price of market-provided services is determined by:

$$P_3 = P_3(P_m,H/I), \quad (5)$$

where P_m is the cost in the market and H/I reflects the extra difficulty that households with health problems or physical impairments may have in making arrangements with vendors.

The price of publicly provided (P_4) services is exogenous because it is defined by program rules. It is important to note that, in reality, the household faces a single supply curve composed of the relevant segments (the lowest price for a given Q) of each of the four schedules described. The resultant supply curve may be highly discontinuous. Since these intricacies cannot be determined, the simplification of including all four prices, without specifying the range over which each is "operable," has been adopted.

Further, because we cannot actually observe most of the prices, it is necessary to utilize a reduced-form model. So substituting supply equations for the price terms in the demand function, and relating the availability of publicly provided services to Y yields:

$$D = D(Y,A,r,HH,SS,H/I,C,N,SI,D_{t-1},NH,Z,P_m,M) \quad (6)$$

The reduced-form specification, while serviceable, has its limitations. In particular, for variables effecting both demand and supply, the estimated coefficients will embody both effects. Four variables in the present model—HH, H/I, Y, and SS—are in this category. On the other hand, the coefficients for the majority of the variables can be given unambiguous interpretations.

A Dynamic Model

The static formulation just presented serves as a useful introduction. It is severely limited, however, as a vehicle for elucidating the housing adjustment process, because it fails to address the major shortcoming of the prior work on in-place adjustments — its non-dynamic character. The most thorough discussion of housing adjustments has been in the context of the decision to relocate. Since the general logic is the same for both in-place adjustments and those accomplished through relocation, a brief review of this work is essential.

Researchers have been remarkably consistent in viewing the household's decision to move locally as resulting from its perception that it will benefit from relocating.[7] Somewhat more precisely, the household is seen as perceiving its current dwelling as not well-suited to its needs and then making the actual decision to move based on the superiority of other housing options, after allowing for the difference in cost between the two units as well as the costs of relocating. The gains in satisfaction over future years from living in the new dwelling are appropriately discounted when compared to the costs associated with the switch.

This simple argument shelters two rather distinct conceptual approaches to considering the local mobility process. The first approach, originally stated by Rossi (1955) and later by Speare et al. (1974), views the household as dissatisfied in some way with its current unit. And it is this "stress" that produces the impetus for moving. The concept of dissatisfaction has not been tightly defined, although it does have a ready intuitive appeal. Numerous empirical studies of mobility have been completed which have employed this general paradigm, with "dissatisfaction" operationalized by direct measures — opinions of households about their homes and neighborhoods — and with proxies measuring putative changes in housing needs due to changes in incomes, households composition, and other factors.[8]

Possibly the most elaborate formulation of this approach was by MacMillan (1980). She postulated the mobility decision as resulting from a process involving four distinct decision phases: the household's perception of dissatisfaction with its present housing situation; a willingness or predisposition of the household to move; the decision to undertake an active search for a new unit; and, lastly, given the information on available options, the decision about relocating. Estimating this four step model with data from the Housing Allowance Demand Experiment, she found reasonable support for this conceptualization.

Economists have pursued a different line of argument and empirical work. The central difference is that they have attempted to attach more exact measurement to the concept of "housing disequilibrium." The standard practice has been to define the equilibrium bundle of housing services for a given household type (specified in terms of income, position in the life cycle, and premove tenure) as that which similar but recently moving households have chosen on average.[9] This is expressed in terms of differences in the rent between the current and equilibrium units. In regression models explaining mobility decisions the difference in rents is included as a key independent variable.

This approach has recently been developed one step further by introducing the concept of equivalent consumer's surplus. This surplus is defined as the amount of additional income that would make the household as well off with its initial housing consumption as it would be in its new, more preferred unit. As in the other approaches, the household is posited to make the decision to move based on the net gain from moving. Here the net gain from moving is the present value of the future stream of the equivalent consumer's surplus over the expected length of stay in the new unit, less the costs associated with mobility. Models of this type were estimated by Cronin (1980), once more exploiting the rich data base from the Housing Allowance Demand Experiment.

Reschovsky (1983) has used this methodology in studying the potential benefits of moving by the elderly. Analyzing data from the Panel Study of Income Dynamics, he found that the potential benefits to the elderly of moving are generally larger than for the nonelderly, i.e., that the elderly are further from their "housing equilibrium" than their more youthful counterparts.

Whereas the "dissatisfaction" models suffer from fuzziness in defining the concept of disequilibrium, one must be equally skeptical about economists' implementation of their more precise formulation. In particular, the flaw comes in defining the equilibrium housing situation as that of households who have occupied a unit for a year or less. This implies an amazing degree of myopia on the part of recent movers, especially when one considers the very substantial transactions costs associated with finding and moving to a new unit. This definition of equilibrium could mean, for example, that a young childless couple would not move to a large single family dwelling in anticipation of having a family over the next several years.[10]

Thus, one can think of households having a desired, equilibrium housing bundle, Y^*, toward which they are adjusting. Partial and sequential adjustments presumably can be observed by those making in-place changes. Each of these changes is due to prior or contemporaneous changes in the factors that determine the demand for housing services enumerated above. So, differences between Y^* and Y are due to changes in the vector of exogenous factors, which we can denote as ΔX. One can anticipate that the effects of many changes will only be evident with the passage of time. That is, an adjustment occurs after the ΔX reaches some critical value.

The general dynamic formulation of the model can be written as: $P(d) = a (Y_t^* - Y_{t-1}) = f (C_{t_0}, X_t, X_{t-1}, X_{t-2} \ldots X_{t_0})$, where P(d) is the probability that a particular adjustment is made (similar to probability of relocating estimated in the mobility literature). t_0 is the beginning of the observation period and t is the end. C_{t_0} is the condition of the dwelling at the start of the period. The independent variables are expressed as their values for each period rather than as changes from the base period or previous period for convenience. In this case ΔY would be the change in level of repair activity undertaken by the household. A lower level of repairs (i.e., $\Delta Y < 0$) might be desirable in responses to declining income, i.e., $X_{t-1} < X_{t-2} < X_{t-3}$. On the other hand, a higher level of repairs ($\Delta Y > 0$) might be needed because of an increase in the depreciation of major components such as the roof or water heater needing replacement.

Specified in this way, the estimated model will provide insights on the length of time between a change in a determinant and the repair decision, as well as whether the effect of the change increases or decreases with time. None of the analyses of repairs and maintenance activities completed to date have employed a dynamic specification.

At the same time, Aquilar and Sandelin (1984) have estimated models of the probability of owner-occupants relocating which employ time series data for each household on income and demographic variables. While some of the lag structures estimated are statistically significant, the coefficients exhibit large year-to-year swings in magnitude and even sign; hence one has little confidence in the specific patterns estimated. Overall then, there is little guidance from the existing literature on the proper structure of dynamic relationships of housing adjustments.[11]

Implications

After considering the various issues raised in this section as well as the data available for this analysis, we have decided on three basic characteristics of the models to be estimated. The first is to use the reduced form model (Equation 6) because the prices of the dependent variable in which we are interested are not observable and, even if they were, we have little theoretical guidance on the expected form of the supply schedules.[12] The second is to employ the binary, probability formulation—i.e., will an adjustment be made over some period or not—that characterizes the mobility studies. As discussed below, this is a much more serviceable specification for several of the housing adjustments under analysis.

Third, we are not employing the explicit disequilibrium formulation favored by economists in their mobility analysis, e.g., how far are the attributes of the household or the unit from their equilibrium values? The principal reasons for this are that no credible equilibrium values can be defined and the measurement problems for proxy variables would be extremely difficult. We have already commented on the problems of viewing recently relocating households as being currently in equilibrium. Likewise, trying to define some younger household or some household making a recent adjustment as having a housing arrangement that is the equilibrium one for another household is fraught with multiple issues of comparability between the households. All in all, we find the explicit measurement of disequilibrium conceptually attractive but empirically impractical to implement.

HOUSING ADJUSTMENTS

In this section we extend the discussion beyond "repairs" and elaborate on the four types of in-place housing adjustments enumerated in the first chapter: modifications of the unit to facilitate its use by family members with a physical impairment; changing the use of rooms to accommodate evolving living arrangements, particularly those associated with activity limitations; renting one or more rooms to nonfamily members; and, improving or depreciating the unit through maintenance and investment activity. For each type of adjustment we discuss what may typically be involved, review what we know about what causes such adjustments to be made, and then comment on issues appropriate to the model just described.

Dwelling Modifications

One way for households to adjust to having a member who experiences an activity limitation is to modify the unit, so as to make discharging daily activities easier for the impaired person. (Another way is to provide compensating personal services, either by family members or from outside of the household.) It is common to picture the dwelling modifications involved as an assortment of grab bars, eliminated thresholds, and the installation of wheelchair ramps. The variety of adjustments is much larger, as shown by the listing in Table 2.1. The list includes features to aid the visually and hearing impaired and those with difficulty grasping as well as those with problems getting about. Table 2.1 also shows the number and percentage of elderly headed (over age 64) households with a member with health problems or activity limitations who are residing in units with some special feature.

Overall, only about 10% of these households reside in such units. Not surprisingly, the most frequent modification is the addition of generally inexpensive and easy-to-install extra handrails and grab

TABLE 2.1

DWELLINGS OCCUPIED BY ELDERLY-HEADED HOUSEHOLDS
WITH AT LEAST ONE MEMBER WITH HEALTH OR MOBILITY PROBLEMS

Modification	Number of Dwellings (in thousands)	Percent of Dwellings
Extra handrails or grab bars	568	6.6
Sink, faucet, cabinet adjustments	103	1.2
Wall socket or light switch adaptations	103	1.2
Elevators or lift chairs	69	0.8
Specifically equipped telephone	69	0.8
Ramps	60	0.7
Extra wide doors or hallways	60	0.7
Door handles instead of knobs	26	0.3
Bathroom designed for wheel chair use	26	0.3
Door handles instead of knobs	26	0.3
Bathroom designed for wheelchair use	26	0.3
Flashing lights	26	0.3
Raised lettering or braille	9	0.1
Push bars on doors	9	0.1
Other features	163	1.9

Total Number of Dwellings With at Least One Modification	886	10.3
Total Number of Dwellings (in thousands)	8,600[a]	

a. Figures do not add to total since not all dwellings have modifications and some report more than one modification.

Source: Tabulations of Annual Housing Survey, 1978, reported in Struyk-Zais (1982), Table 2, p. 7.

bars. One analyst has estimated that about one million additional elderly headed households live in situations in which modifications are very likely needed.[13]

There has been one comprehensive analysis of the demand for the special features by the elderly who head their own households. In this study Struyk (1982) employed the 1978 national Annual Housing Survey, which included a special supplement on health status and dwelling modifications. The study applied bivariate and multivariate analytic techniques to dichotomous (0/1) dependent variables for some of the modifications listed in Table 2.1. The major findings about what factors are important in determining whose units are modified are as follows.[14]

Tenure

Simple tabulations on renters and homeowners do not show significant differences which one might have expected. Owners have the legal right to modify their own homes, but renters must generally convince landlords to install special features, or search for a unit that has them. The results do indicate that the specific factors associated with living in a modified unit differ for renters and owners. Still, just having information on tenure does not lead to straight forward conclusions about the probability of living in an adapted dwelling.

Income

Surprisingly, household income was generally found *not* to be a significant determinant of a household having a special feature in its unit. In only one case — bathroom modifications for homeowners — was income significant in explaining its presence. Overall, the results do not suggest that income is a persistent constraint to living in a unit with special features, although the analysis lacked full information on a household's asset position, which may affect whose units are modified.

Severity of Health and Mobility Problems

Several dimensions of severity were tested, including the share of family members with such problems and the occurrence of more than one problem per family member. Such factors were consistently and strongly related to the presence of special features. Activity limitations, more than health problems, were especially good indicators. The presence of someone who needs a special appliance and/or personal assistance to get around was also highly predictive. Contrary to expectations, however, difficulty in using the sink, faucets or cabinets was *not* related to the presence of special features for handling this problem. Overall, though, the general picture is one of a strong relationship between severity and the presence of special features.

Household Type and Position in Household

Surprising results were also observed here. Whether or not the impaired person lives alone or is a member of a multiperson household is not especially important in affecting the probability of living in a modified unit. There was, however, evidence that position in the household for those not living alone *does* matter: special features are more likely to be present if the *head* needs mechanical assistance or both mechanical and personal assistance, than if another household member does. Unfortunately, the data did not permit more detailed testing as to why this should be the case.

Price of Special Features

In this part of the analysis wage rates were used to estimate the a real variation in the price of modifying a unit, because it was assumed that the cost of materials is generally comparable across geographical areas. The importance of price measured in this way varied, proving significant in some cases, and insignificant in others. Generally, however, the higher the "price," the less likely households were to live in specially equipped dwellings.

The present analysis will also examine whether individual modifications have been made. Use of the 0/1 formulation—no change vs. change—is especially apt here, where continuous measurements of the extent of changes are particularly difficult to construct.

Changing Room Use

Another way of coping with activity limitations on the part of household members is to redefine the purpose for which rooms are used. Such changes presumably are most frequent where stairs make using the whole unit quite difficult or impossible for the impaired member. Thus, we observe the situation in which a first floor den has been converted into a bedroom, both to make it easier for the caregiver to attend to the disabled family member and to make it possible for the disabled person to be included more in the daily routine than if he spent most of his days in a second floor bedroom. Sometimes more radical room changes are necessary. A common example here is the installation of a bathroom on the first floor (perhaps converting a pantry), so that the person with moderate difficulty negotiating stairs does not have to do so more than once or twice a day.

While those familiar with the living arrangements of elderly homeowners think of such adjustments as quite commonplace, there is remarkably little documentation of the incidence of such changes and only limited understanding of the role (or potential role) which such shifts may play in enabling the elderly to remain in their homes. As far as we know, there are no data presently available, even from case studies, on this point. [15]

Again, the binary formulation is appropriate. We had hoped to give changes involving bathrooms and sleeping arrangements special attention; but, as discussed in Chapter 4, the incidence of such changes in our sample is very low. In general, since the likelihood of change is expected to be especially sensitive to the configuration of the unit (e.g., location of the bathroom), it would be important to control for this factor.

Renting a Room

While individual homeowners have rented out rooms for as long as we can remember, there has been a recent surge of interest in room renting as an element of the housing policy for the elderly. [16] One suspects that the possibilities for room rental by the elderly has risen in the past 25 years as higher post-retirement incomes and a greater incidence of homeownership has produced a large number of "over housed" elderly couples and individuals. Some policy analysts see home sharing or room renting as a way to help those elderly who wish to remain in their homes do so by alleviating income problems and increasing the within-home supportive services available to the family members.

In the past few years, in addition to much policy discussion, [17] several case studies of room-renting by elderly headed households have been conducted. We rely here on findings reported in Schreter (1983), Howe et al. (1984), and Pritchard (1983). All three find that those sharing their homes are motivated to do so by the need for additional income and some supportive services. Interestingly, most "home sharers" are women in the 55-70 age group; most do not have serious activity limitations. The overwhelming attraction for "room seekers" to live in such arrangements is the low rent. Experience on the amount of services provided by room seekers to home sharers appears to vary sharply among programs, precluding any general statement. Importantly, Pritchard's data, which cover a 12-month period, show that many of these sharing arrangements only last a few months; this is confirmed by the experience documented by Howe et al.

As far as we know, there are no reliable national data on this phenomenon. Most surveys which inventory household members only ascertain if a person is not related to the head of the house, not if the person is also paying rent for a room to live with the balance of household.[18]

The apparent episodic nature of house sharing arrangements—at least those associated with "matching" programs—suggest the need to examine as long a history as possible for each household under study. Again, the binary formulation seems appropriate.

Maintenance and Investment

The opening section of this chapter discussed the determinants of dwelling and investment decisions in substantial detail. In light of this, we have elected at this point to make only a few general observations on these decisions. In particular, the forces driving these decisions can be divided into two broad groups: maximization of the rate of return on the unit, and maximization of the "use value" of the unit to its current occupants.

Typically, when one thinks about the investment motive he imagines such cases as the household deciding whether modernizing the kitchen will result in an increase in the value of the house in excess of the rehabilitation cost. The primary consideration here is the trend in property values in the neighborhood and the position of the value of the home in question compared to others. While many decisions are of this type, including the amount of routine maintenance and refurbishing to conduct, at least one class of decisions differs significantly: low-income elderly who have become "locked in" to their home because of the high perceived out-of-pocket cost of moving to a smaller owner-occupied or rental unit.[19] When proper up-keep of their home would require such households to sacrifice consumption of needed things, they deliberately decide to follow a program of under maintenance, i.e., of allowing the asset value of their home to decline. In effect, they are generating income for these other purchases by drawing down on their home equity — by neglecting upkeep expenditures. One can readily imagine that the cost of maintenance is higher for those unable to do it themselves. Hence, those especially likely to be undermaintaining are low-income households, women living alone or a couple with an impaired member.

The second determinant — enhanced use-value of the unit — can result in higher levels of investment in housing, although still perhaps with inadequate maintenance. For cases in which a person lives alone or in a household where the amount of personal assistance available is limited, the onset of serious activity limitations may well call forth changes to the unit to permit the individual to continue to occupy it. These could be large expenditures, such as installing a bathroom on the ground floor of a two-story home. Because such unit modifications would be relative few, it is likely that for the undermaintaining household they would appear as a sharp deviation from the regular pattern of expenditures on unit maintenance and investment, if one were able to observe the household's expenditures over an extended time horizon.

In Table 2.2 we present the most reliable national figures available on repair activity by elderly homeowners. These data from a Census survey which returns to the same households for several quarters to obtain this information.[20] The figures in the table are for two calendar quarters, so they might be doubled to get the upper-limit values to the percentage of households undertaking such activities. It is clear that even with this adjustment there is a substantial minority of households not undertaking any repairs or improvements to their home over the course of the year. While surely not all of these households are disinvesting, this does point to a less uni-

TABLE 2.2

Percentage of Homeowners Undertaking Repairs or Improvement to Their Dwellings, in a Quarter During the First and Third Quarters of 1977

	Head 65 Years or Older			Heads under Age 65		
	Any Expenditure	Repairs	Improvement	Any Expenditure	Repairs	Improvements
Income						
Under $5,000	15	14	1	23	13	6
$5,000-$9,999	32	24	11	32	24	12
$10,000-$14,999	34	27	9	37	29	16
$15,000 and over	32	28	9	42	31	20
Year Dwelling Built						
After 1960	22	13	6	35	23	17
1950-1959	23	20	5	33	23	17
1940-1949	29	23	6	31	24	13
Before 1940	23	20	6	36	27	16
Location						
Inside SMSA	27	21	3	38	29	17
Outside SMSA	22	19	5	34	25	16
Location by Income						
Inside SMSAs						
Under $5,000	13	a	a	21	a	a
$ 5,000-$9,999	31			42		
$10,000-$14,999	37			38		
$15,000 and over	31			42		
Outside SMSAs						
Under $5,000	14	a	a	24	a	a
$ 5,000-$9,999	34			30		
$10,000-$14,999	26			35		
$15,000 and over	36			41		

Source: Special tabulations from the U.S. Bureau of the Census, Survey of Residential Repairs and Alternations, Series C-50, reported in Struyk-Soldo (1980), Table 4-1.

a Sample sizes too small for reliable calculations.

33

versal pattern of dwelling upkeep activity than might have been thought.

The analysis of housing maintenance and investment expenditures to date has been rather limited, mostly consisting of analyses of data for a single year using a fairly restricted set of explanatory variables.[21] The most comprehensive of these was by Struyk and Soldo (1980, Chapter 4). They analyzed the determinants of the probability of elderly homeowners making maintenance repairs to their dwellings and the determinants of the choice among three "suppliers": themselves, friends or family members living outside of the home, and hired contractors. The data were from a special survey of about 1,500 elderly homeowners in seven locations sponsored by the Department of Housing and Urban Development (HUD). The data set was relatively rich, including information on dwelling condition, physical limitations of household members, neighborhood conditions, and the extent to which children not living with their parents were providing support to their parents. On the other hand, it omitted some important variables such as formal support services received, and had weak information on others. Additionally, the elderly were asked to recall repair activity over the prior two years—an extraordinarily long time. In view of these limitations, the analysis was considered exploratory.

Among the suggestive findings of this work are the following:

— An elderly homeowner is more likely to do the repair himself if it is a husband-wife household; a higher income also increases this probability. The likelihood falls sharply with advanced age and mobility limitations.
— The probability of a family member or friend making at least one repair increases as the number of persons visiting the elderly person/couple increases. The fact that this likelihood declines with increasing income suggests the elderly rely on family and friends more often when financially constrained to do so. Surprisingly, age and mobility impairments have little effect on repair activity when friends are making the repairs.
— The probability of the elderly hiring workmen or contractors to make repairs is positively related to income, being a nonhusband/wife household, and being older. The housing quality

coefficients suggest that hired labor is used more often when units are in good condition, a phenomenon possibly related to past household income.

A second related study, also reported in Struyk-Soldo (1980, Chapter 5), attempted to fill in some of the gap in the prior analysis which resulted from a lack of information on support services. Here, the relationship was estimated among an index of housing upkeep and a series of determinants, including the receipt of help with heavy housework. One hypothesis was that this type of support service would influence the ability of the household to maintain its home, and thus be reflected in dwelling condition. The sample for this analysis was 5,900 elderly headed households (both owners and renters) in the 1974 wave of the Survey of the Low-Income and Disabled (SLIAD). Multiple regression analysis was used as the estimation technique, but owing to specification limitations, the analysis was again considered exploratory. Important findings include the following:

- Higher incomes and more assets are consistently associated with fewer dwelling defects.
- Units occupied by a widow or a married couple will have fewer defects than units occupied by other types of households.
- Physical impairments by homeowner respondents are associated with more dwelling defects.
- Receipt of the services delivered—meals, visiting nurse, or help finding a place to live—is associated with higher-quality units for urban and rural renters; by contrast, receiving assistance with housekeeping improves dwelling quality only for urban renters. No effects for homeowners were found, possibly owing to the very small number receiving such services.

These various findings form the basis for a number of hypotheses tested in the multivariate analysis in Chapter 5.

Of particular interest is the stability of repair activity over time, i.e., are some households consistently disinvesting? This is addressed in the binary formulation framework by assigning a value of one to cases in which, for example, a household is consistently in the lowest quartile of the distribution of maintenance and investment expenditures. Several such specifications are tested in Chapter 5, permitting us to take advantage of the greater (continuous) information on these activities but still within the basic model framework.

Related Adjustments

The discussion thus far may have implied that these different types of adjustments occur rather independently of each other. In reality, these different adjustments may well be related. A change in room usage may well require some modifications to the room. Likewise, carrying out any dwelling modification should show up in the cost of repairs and investments; and, if it is a change like making a closet into a bathroom, it will also be classified as a room modification. Similarly, the decision to take in a roomer may mean both room usage changes and investments to make some unit modifications to insure the minimum level of privacy. In short, the household makes it adjustment decisions as a group. Of course, in response to changes in household composition, health status, and the like, these decisions may be repeated at several points over the years with adjustments occurring in clusters.

CAUSAL FACTORS

This section provides some further discussion on the effects which the independent variables enumerated in the exposition of the conceptual model may have on the type and extent of in-place housing adjustments made by the elderly. The added detail both enriches the conceptual model and provides essential background for the analysis in Chapters 4 and 5.

Table 2.3 gives a summary of the anticipated affects which these factors would have on the four types of housing adjustments being considered. Below, we look at each factor separately, first expanding on the thinking behind the hypotheses and then presenting some germane information about the factor itself.

TABLE 2.3

Summary of Expected Effects of Causal Factors on the Probability of Different Types of Housing Adjustments

Causal Factors	Prob. of dwelling Modification	Prob. of Having Boarders Present	Prob. of Room Usage Change	Prob. of Extensive Repairs and Investments
A. Strong economic position	raises P[a]	lowers P	raises P	lowers P
B. Activity limitations	raises P	lowers P	raises P	lowers P
C. Social support/interaction	raises P	ambiguous	raises P	raises P
D. Help with activities of daily living	lowers P	raises P	lowers P	raises P
E. More supportive living arrangements	raises P	lowers P	ambiguous	raises P
F. 1. Poor dwelling condition	--[b]	--	--	raises P
2. Multi-story unit w. upstairs bath only	raises P	--	raises P	--
G. Poor neighborhood conditions	lowers P	--	--	lowers P
H. Respondent intends to move	lowers P	--	lowers P	ambiguous

a. P is probability.
b. A dash indicates that the factor is not expected to directly effect this type of adjustment.

Economic Position

Clearly high incomes and strong asset positions make it easier for households to make various kinds of adjustments. They can simply afford to make more changes that will enhance the quality of their daily lives. Hence, dwelling modifications should be more common, and unit upkeep more extensive. Similarly, a weak economic position will encourage disinvestment in the dwelling.

There is one offsetting factor present, however, that should be noted: those with greater economic resources can also afford to purchase more personal services, such as maid or personal assistance help; to the extent that these services are purchased, they will reduce the likelihood of compensating dwelling modifications being undertaken by households with a physically impaired member.

Additionally, it is our hypothesis that generating increased income is a very important factor in the decision to take a boarder into a person's home. Hence, we expect that those in stronger economic circumstances will be less likely to have a boarder present.

Having made these points, some caveats are appropriate. First, the desirable definition of a household's economic position is quite broad, including actual cash income, the imputed return on nonincome producing assets, particularly home equity, and the value of in-kind transfer such as Medicare. Danzinger et al. (1984) show, for example, that employing such a definition, along with corrections for household size, raises the ratio of elderly income to nonelderly income from .49 to .90 in 1973. Naturally, the more comprehensive measure will also effect the ranking of the economic positions of the elderly among themselves.[22] Importantly, a broader definition of income more closely approximates the idea of a household's permanent income – or its "normal" level – over its lifetime. Income measured in this way is relevant for understanding its current circumstances, such as living in an expensive home but having a comparatively low-income level.

Second, the dynamics of income flows surrounding retirement need to be recognized. A recent paper by Fox (1984) documents the shift in income levels and composition accompanying retirement, using data from the Retirement History Survey. His analysis gives a picture of the situation for households retiring in the mid-1970s.

This analysis used a cash definition of income that is less comprehensive than that just suggested as desirable. Among the study's principal findings are:

— Married couples had the highest levels of preretirement income but incurred the greatest decrease in income upon entering the Social Security benefit rolls. In real terms, couples lost about a third of their preretirement income (a median of $24,000 in 1982 dollars). Nonmarried women started lower, at $11,000, but lost only a fourth of their income.
— Income composition changed considerably, from almost exclusive reliance on earnings to a mixture of sources, dominated by Social Security and other pension income. For married couples, Social Security and other pension income accounted for 60% of aggregate income, while asset income and earnings each accounted for a 20% share. For nonmarried women the importance of asset income was fractionally lower than for couples, and that of earnings greater.
— Close to half had earned income one or two years after benefit receipt, though in amounts that were only a fraction of their previous levels.
— Persons with low previous income experienced less of a decline in their total income than did those with higher initial income. This finding reflects the progressive structure of Social Security benefits and the greater propensity of low-income beneficiaries to continue working.
— Asset income consisted primarily of interest and dividends, with rental income a distant second except among couples without pensions other than Social Security. The proceeds of private insurance and annuities were almost never received (Fox, 1984, pp. 21-22).

Fox also contrasted the incomes of a set of households just after retirement with their incomes four years later. As might be expected, earnings decrease in importance and the share of households — especially individuals — receiving public assistance rises. Overall, incomes declined about 5% over the period, mostly due to the corrosive effects of high inflation rates during these years.

These figures suggest considerable income shifts for those whose living arrangements did not change over the observation period. (The survey tracked couples and individuals who remained in these statuses over the period.) For those changing marital status—especially couples experiencing death of the husband—the changes are even sharper.[23]

Consequently, knowing the household's economic position before and throughout the period over which one anticipates adjustments to occur is essential to understanding the observed patterns. Moreover, because housing adjustments may occur with an appreciable lag after a reduction in income, a several year income history is highly desirable for the analysis.

Activity Limitations

Housing changes in response to the onset of activity limitations by the person living alone or by one member of a couple is perhaps the most intuitively clear of the causal relationships being considered. The immediacy of the need for change seems obvious. Indeed, holding other factors constant, the expected effects of the presence of a household head or spouse with an activity limitation are to: (a) raise the likelihood of compensating dwelling modifications and room usage changes being made; and, (b) lower the likelihood of repairs and investment to the unit, as there will be fewer "household inputs" available for performing or managing these tasks.

While the effect on the likelihood of having a boarder present is less clear, we believe that it will reduce the likelihood, again on the ground that family will be less able to manage this additional activity if it must provide additional assistance to one of its own members. Still, for a person living alone the effect of an activity limitation, which creates the real need for a modest amount of personal assistance, could be to attract a boarder who whould discharge this function, presumably in exchange for reduced room rent.

What is the incidence of disabilities that might require compensating changes to the residential environment or make taking care of the unit substantially more difficult? Two types of data can be marshalled to address this question. First, there have been a number of tabulations of the number of elderly who need long-term care assistance. While much of the assistance required would be in the form of personnel services, some limitations could be overcome through changes to the unit. Soldo (1983) has used the 1979 National Health Interview Survey data to compute the incidence figures shown in Table 2.4. Overall, about 12% of those over age 65 and 21% of those over 75 are classified as needing home care (see notes to table for definitions). One notable pattern, to which we will return, is that those living alone have lower incidence of need for such care — reflecting the fact that without home care individuals are more likely to be institutionalized, whereas persons with similar problems in other living arrangements have a better chance of remaining in their homes.[24] The high incidence rates for those living with non-relatives or with a relative other than a spouse indicates the intense level of care provided in many of these cases.

The second approach to estimating the need for compensating unit modifications is to count the number of households having a member with an activity limitation which directly interferes with his ability to use the home. Such counts were done using the 1978 Annual Housing Survey data mentioned earlier in this chapter. The percentage of households headed by a person over age 64 found to have a member with an activity limitation is:[25]

Type of Limitation	Percentage
Going in and out of the home	11.2
Getting around inside the dwelling	7.7
Going up and down stairs	16.5
Using equipment in the bathroom or kitchen	5.5
Completely bedridden	1.3

These percentages are not additive because a person may have more than one type of limitation. Still, they suggest that perhaps one household in four has an activity impairment that could be ameliorated through some change to the unit.[26] On the other hand, families may decide to respond to these needs through helping the impaired persons rather than altering the dwelling.

TABLE 2.4

Prevalence Rate Per 1000 Persons Aged 65+ of Need
for Home Care for Selected Characteristics, by Age: 1979[a]

Characteristics	Total	Age 65 - 74	Age 75+
Total	121.0	69.9	211.0
Race			
White	116.0	64.0	207.0
Black	168.0	127.0	245.0
Other	148.0	82.0	320.0
Sex			
Male	91.0	55.3	166.6
Female	141.0	81.1	237.2
Region			
Northeast	129.0	78.0	219.0
North Central	104.0	54.0	188.0
South	130.0	80.0	221.0
West	118.0	62.0	216.0
Place of Residence			
Central City, SMSA	123.0	77.0	204.0
SMSA, not Central City	113.0	64.0	203.0
Rural, nonfarm	132.0	74.0	230.0
Rural, farm	72.0	25.0	164.0
Living Arrangements			
Alone	124.0	77.0	177.0
With Non-Relative	246.0	132.0	392.0
With Spouse	82.0	55.0	163.0
With Other Relative	243.0	134.0	346.0

---

a. A person is defined as needing home care if any of the following
conditions are met: (a) needed or received help or was unable to
perform any of the seven ADL activities (see below); (b) needed or
received help with at least one of the four IADL activities; (c) stayed
in bed all or most of the time; or (d) needed help with a urinary or
bowel device. ADL (activities of daily living) include toileting,
bathing, dressing, eating, transference, incontinence, cutting
toenails. IADL (instrumental activities of daily living) include meal
preparation, shopping, performing chores, and light housework.

Source: Estimates from the 1979 National Health Interview Survey
prepared by Soldo (1983), Figure 1 and Table 2.

Supportive Services

As suggested earlier, one can think of at least three different types of support that will effect the ability of the elderly person to remain in the community and possibly make (or forego) adjustments to his housing situation short of relocating. These are (a) the arrangement in which the person lives, extending from being alone to being in a multiperson household with many "helpers" available; (b) the extent of social interaction with family living outside the household and friends and the support received from these sources; and (c) assistance received from outside the home with tasks of daily living, provided either by family or friends or on a purchased basis. These factors are especially important in this discussion because receipt of such assistance may sharply reduce the need for the kinds of housing adjustments being analyzed.

Although these are listed as separate factors in Table 2.3 and indeed to have discrete identities, their close interrelationship must be acknowledged. As one example, we would expect that those from a rich at-home family environment would pursue social activities outside of the home with less vigor than those living alone, and thus derive less support from such contacts. Similarly, the presence of "helpers" in the home will substitute for help from outside the home, for many types of needed assistance.

It is because of the close relation among these factors that we discuss them as a group. We begin by considering their separate anticipated effects on housing adjustments and then review briefly the current information on the incidence of such supports.[27]

As to household composition one can, in general, array different types of households in terms of the amount of support that they will likely be providing to those present. Living alone is least supportive (with men probably less equipped than women for this life) and living in a household with several adults the most supportive. The central hypothesis is that in more supportive environments there will be less need for changes to the unit to accommodate physical impairments. On the other hand, this same environment means that there are "more hands" available among whom to spread the work (the actual work or the management of it) and more people who may notice problems with the unit and argue for repairs and improvements to be made. Hence, we anticipate (other things the same) for more supportive households to be more active in keeping up their units but less active in modifying them when an impaired household member is present.

There is a general concern in the gerontological literature that with children gone from the family and without daily contact of coworkers provided by employment, the elderly lose important bases for social integration. This may be compounded by declining health and incomes, which can limit the range of activities outside the home that are undertaken. In short, there may be a real tendency for the elderly to become isolated.

The idea behind inclusion of social support/interactions in explaining housing adjustments is that, at least among the elderly, the more active and engaged they are in the community and the more contact they have with their children, then the more likely they are to have the energy level needed to undertake these adjustments, to be more aware of the community's standards for dwelling upkeep, and to draw on others for needed help, even if it is only "technical assistance" or referrals for contractors. Again, of course, these effects are anticipated after holding other causal factors constant.

The probability of taking a boarder is the one type of adjustment for which the effect of social supports is ambiguous. On the one hand, this type of support enhances the ability of the household to overcome the problems of changing the unit, if necessary, and attracting the first boarder. On the other hand, to the extent that a boarder is sought to provide some degree of social support, then the boarder is less necessary if the household receives a high degree of support from other sources.

Since assistance from outside the home with activities of daily living is explicitly to compensate for the types of activity limitations captured by the variables discussed earlier, one expects the effects of this assistance to be systematically in the opposite direction from the effects for the presence of impaired household members. Thus, help of this type lowers the odds of various types of dwelling modifications and raises the odds of a boarder being present and of a high level of repair and maintenance actions being undertaken.

A very substantial amount of research has been done on the type and extent of support services elderly headed households receive.

The task of the next few paragraphs is only to sketch the results of the work. At the outset, though, it is useful to make the distinction between the availability of support services and their actual utilization. A number of studies have examined the presence of potential care providers (or "helpers"), within the person's household or within a certain distance from his home. The assumption is that these available helpers will provide the assistance that is needed. In contrast, utilization moves from potential to actuality. In concept the difference is quite similar to that between need and demand. To use the available services the person needing them must be willing to "pay for them." Of course, the price is generally only expressed in dollars and cents for purchased formal services; rather, price often takes the form of incurring social obligations and acknowledging a lack of competence to others which can be perceived as losing authority or stature. Additionally, the supply of services (the willingness with which informal sources are willing or able to help) is quite sensitive to the intensity and duration of the assistance needed. In practice it appears that there is considerable variance between availability and utilization which makes it valuable to bear the distinction in mind.

We can obtain a good idea of the extent of utilization of support services from all sources from the figures in Table 2.5, which were compiled by Soldo (1983a) from the 1979 National Health Interview Survey. These figures are only for persons classified as needing home care services (following the definition used earlier[28]). They show that only 2.3% of the persons needing services do not receive any. On the other hand, 88% of those receiving services obtain at least some of them from informal sources; indeed, almost 73% obtain them only from informal sources, while 16% receive services from both formal and informal sources. So, the vast majority of the elderly who remain in the community do receive at least some of the support services they need, and most of these come from family members and friends.

Soldo analyzed these data further by estimating a logit model determining the probability of a person in need of services obtaining them from a formal source. The figures in Table 2.6 are probabili-

TABLE 2.5

Percentage Distribution of Respondents Age 65 and Over
In Need of Home Care by Service Use Patterns
(percents)

Informal Service Receipt	Formal Service Receipt [a]		Total
	Receives Services	Does not Receive Services	
Receives Services from the Informal Support Network	15.9 (227)[b]	72.6 (1039)	88.5 (1266)
Does not Receive Services from the Informal Support Network	9.2 (132)	2.3 (33)	11.5 (165)
Total	25.1 (359)	74.9 (1072)	100.0 (1431)

a. See note to Table 2.4 for definition of "home care" population.

b. Sample size.

Source: Estimates from the Home Care Supplement to the 1979 National
         Health Interview Survey, reported in Soldo (1983a), Table 2.

ties of persons with varying levels of need and in different living
arrangements receiving formal services. Two patterns are starkly
evident: as the intensity of need increases, the likelihood of obtaining these services accelerates; and, the incidence of receipt of formal services is consistently higher for those living alone and those
living with nonrelatives, compared with those living with their
spouse or other relatives.[29]

Living arrangements are clearly an important determinant of the
source and extent of support services received. Cantor (1979) reports that nearly 90% of informally provided services come from
family members, most from within the home. The figures on the
higher incidence of formal services used by those living alone cited
above are consistent with the absence support provided by other
adults in the home. So, too, is the finding that rates of institutionalization are higher among those not currently married (most of
whom live alone) than for those living in more supportive arrange-

TABLE 2.6

Probability of Formal Service Receipt by Type
of Living Arrangement and Need,
for Those With Informal Supports[1]

Type of Need	Probability of Formal Service Receipt Type of Living Arrangement			
	Alone	With Nonrelative	With Spouse	With Other Relative
IADL Need Only	.17	.31	.08	.04
ADL Need Only	.27	.44	.14	.08
Medical Need Only	.31	.50	.17	.09
ADL & IADL Need	.44	.62	.26	.14
ADL & Medical Need	.63	.79	.43	.27
ADL, IADL & Medical Needs	.78	.61	.44	.44
All Types of Needs & Incontinence Problems	.86	.93	.74	.58
All Types of Need & Incontinence and Supervision Problems	⁰.90	.95	.81	.68

1. Logistic function (Probability (P) = 1/1 + e^{-xb}) evaluated for white women residing in central citites with annual family incomes of $5000 - 9999 (in 1978 dollars) who did not participate in Medicaid in 12 months preceding interview.

Source: Soldo (1983a); results of logit model are in Table 3, while the estimates shown here are in Table 4.

ments, after having controlled for economic, health status, and other conditions (Weissert & Scanlon, 1983, p.16).[30] More generally, those living alone show a variety of disadvantages in well-being compared to married couples (Lawton, Moss & Kleban, 1984).

Logically, it would seem that living arrangements also strongly effect the amount of social contact a person may have. Multiperson households can provide much of the needed interaction and support that those living alone must seek elsewhere. Interestingly, studies to date indicate that the elderly respond to changes in their living arrangements by developing the necessary compensating relationships. A recent study by Kohen (1983), for example, documents that the elderly widowed are not more isolated than the elderly married and that elderly women have some advantage over elderly men in their ability to develop or maintain social relationships.[31]

Acknowledging the importance of living arrangements and supports, we still can ask who actually provides informal support services to the elderly. It may be useful in this regard to briefly look at the extent of the availability of family members for providing these services. Table 2.7 reports on the proximity of children and siblings for a sample of elderly living in a mid-western metropolitan area. These figures show that 92% of the persons sampled had at least one surviving child or sibling and 79% had at least one survivor living within 50 miles of his home. These figures are quite consistent with others which generally paint a picture of widespread availability of potential helpers.[32]

As to actual utilization, survey results presented by Stoller and Earl (1983) provide a comprehensive perspective.[33] Some of their results, summarized in Table 2.8, show the percentage of those elderly who classified themselves as being unable to perform particular activities without assistance who receive the needed assistance

TABLE 2.7

Proximity of Surviving Children and Siblings for Elderly
Persons in the Wichita Area, 1981
(percentage of persons with each number of survivors)

Number	Total Surviving	Within 50 Miles
0	8	21
1	12	31
2	17	20
3	14	12
4	14	7
5	11	4
6	24	5
Total	100	100

Source: Hays (1984), Table 3, p. 152.

from various sources. Data are given in the table for five activities. Consistent with the figures presented earlier, formal providers are relatively unimportant; and few persons do without essential services.[34] Spouses and daughters bear the primary burden of assisting. Other relatives and friends provide significant but distinctly less important levels of aid and are about equally important on average.[35] Despite the dominance of family support indicated, it is worth noting that such providers tend to experience serious fatigue when providing care over extended periods; in some case formal services become more important, but in others the result is institutionalization.[36]

In brief, there is a host of living arrangement and supportive service factors which will strongly effect the type and extent of housing adjustments made. These factors are heavily interrelated, which suggests that one be quite cautious in assigning a causal role to any individual factor identified in our statistical work as being important.

TABLE 2.8

Prevalence of Helpers of Elderly Persons
Reporting They Definitely Could Not Do a Task by Themselves [a,b]
(percentages)

	Task				
Helper	Preparing Food	Shopping	Bathing	Light Chores	Heavy Chores
none	—	—	10	33	—
spouse	37	30	25	24	26
daughter	35	40	42	31	38
son	5	9	12	3	5
other relative	13	14	7	7	13
friend	9	13	5	3	6
formal provider	6	—	9	10	6

a. Sample of 753 elderly persons residing in a metro-areas of a 17-county region of northeastern New York.
b. For the daughter, son, and other relative categories of helpers it is not clear whether they live with the person assisted or not.

Source: Stoller and Earl (1983), Table 2, p. 66.

Dwelling Attributes

Two types of dwelling characteristics are germane to this discussion. One is the condition of the unit at the start of the observation period. To the extent that it is in poor repair, it will have a greater requirement for higher levels of maintenance and investment than other units. Whether the household responds to this is another question, since disrepair may signal an intentional program of disinvestment or an inability to make repairs. Aside from the influence on maintenance levels, it seems doubtful that unit condition would effect the incidence of other types of adjustment.[38]

These are clear patterns in the presence of dwelling deficiencies among the elderly homeowners, some of which are highlighted in the figures in Table 2.9 from the Annual Housing Survey. For one thing, elderly headed households with income below the poverty level live in units with higher rates of deficiencies than their more affluent counterparts. Also, husband-wife households live in the best units, as indicated by lack of these deficiencies at all income levels, with persons living alone next, and other types of elderly headed households in the worst housing.[38] A third pattern (not shown in the table) is that these households with a person with activity limitations have a higher incidence of living in units with some deficiency than do other households. Using a somewhat different set of deficiency measures than those shown in the notes to the table, Newman (1985) found these rates to be 17% and 10%, respectively, for households with an impaired member and other households. All of this suggests that the reasons for the presence of dwelling deficiencies are complicated and that the presence of such deficiencies may signal an equally rich variety of circumstances.

The second type of unit attribute that could effect the likelihood of various adjustments is its configuration. To the degree that key rooms — kitchen, bathroom and bedrooms — are located exclusively on different floors in the original design, the greater then odds that room use changes and extensive dwelling modifications will be undertaken by households with physically impaired members. Among single-family homes at one extreme is the single-floor, ranch-style home with all rooms on one level; at the other is the center-hall colonial in which the kitchen is on the ground floor and the bath-

TABLE 2.9

Rates of Housing Deficiencies for Elderly Homeowners: 1976
(percentages)

	plumbing	kitchen	sewage	heat	maintenance
Household Type and Income					
Husband-wife					
below poverty	9.01	4.01	.67[b]	.57[b]	3.05
poverty to twice poverty	1.97	.85	.38[b]	.27[b]	1.27
over twice poverty	.57	.28[b]	.19[b]	.16[b]	.83
Total	1.85	.84	.30	.24	1.19
Single persons					
below poverty	10.50	5.77	.24[b]	.82[b]	4.61
poverty to twice poverty	3.50	1.45	.45[b]	.28[b]	1.69
over twice poverty	1.23	.73[b]	.00[b]	.19[b]	1.65
Total	4.55	2.32	.25	.39	2.43
Other					
below poverty	11.65	6.10	.27[b]	.81[b]	9.20
poverty to twice poverty	6.83	4.27	.38[b]	.94[b]	3.44
over twice poverty	2.87	1.05[b]	.35[b]	.62[b]	3.34
Total	5.94	3.10	.34[b]	.75[b]	4.61

Deficiencies[a]

a.

Variable Name	Description
Plumbing	Unit either lacks complete plumbing facilities or household must share their use.
Kitchen	Unit either lacks a complete kitchen or household must share their use.
Sewage	One or more of the following three services was unavailable or completely unusable for six or more hours at least three times during the past ninety days: (1) running water, (2) sewage system, (3) toilet.
Heat	The heating system was completely unusable for six or more hours at least three times during the past winter.
Maintenance	Two or more of the following four conditions exist: (1) leaking roof, (2) substantial cracks or holes in walls and ceiling, (3) holes in floors, (4) broken plaster or peeling paint in areas larger than 1 square foot.

b. Sample size to small for estimate to be reliable.

Source: Struyk-Soldo (1980), Table 3-6.

room and bedrooms are on the second level. We would anticipate more room usage changes and modifications for the center-hall colonial.

There is surprisingly little information from national surveys about the arrangement of rooms within a unit. One national study shows that among 1-4 unit structures 70% are single-floor units, exclusive of basements and attics.[39] This suggests that about half of the single unit structures are so configured. The data collected as part of this study for areas in seven cities, described in the next chapter, show that 35% of these owner-occupied units are more than a single story. In terms of the arrangement of rooms, an important issue is the extent to which both a bedroom and bath are on the first floor, thereby eliminating trips up and down steps in order for those with severe mobility impairments to be involved in the everyday life of the household. Our survey data shows the following percentage of multifloor units with various arrangements on the first floor:

bedroom but not bath present	6
bath but no bedroom	28
both bedroom and bath present	31

These figures indicate that more of housing stock may already be potentially rather more accommodating to those with mobility limitations than might otherwise be thought.

Poor Neighborhood Conditions

Every homeowner is concerned to some degree that he not "overinvest" in his home — not make improvements to the unit that will cost him more than he will be able to obtain when the unit is sold, after having made appropriate allowance for the use-value he will obtain from the improvements while he lives there. Neighborhood conditions are a key determinant of house values in this country.[40] Thus, neighborhood conditions are expected to effect those adjustments that require significant investment in the unit: making extensive physical modifications to accommodate the impaired member and general improvement expenditures. The worse the neighborhood, the less investment is expected.

Since objective, direct indicators on neighborhood conditions are lacking on a national basis, we do not provide documentation of these circumstances for the elderly. It is worth noting, however, that it does appear that the elderly do reside in neighborhoods with more potential problems – a higher rate of low value and low rent units and single-parent families – than do households headed by a younger person.[41] In our analysis, however, it is the variation in neighborhood conditions, and their impact on housing investment, which is of interest.

NOTES

1. Parts of this model are presented, for example, in Struyk-Soldo (1980), Chapter 4.

2. In recent years, economists have noted that housing in general is a differentiated good, in both demand and supply. The principal distinctions have to do with structural attributes of dwellings and the characteristics of the neighborhoods in which they are located. This is thoroughly exposited in Straszheim (1975), and Kain and Quigley (1975). More recent econometric analysis includes work by Follain and Malpezzi (1980).

3. D_{t-1} is total repair activity in the previous period.

4. One might argue that a countervailing effect would be economies of scale from doing several jobs at the same time. In fact, since most tasks are quite discrete, the size of such economies would appear to be small in general.

5. Other factors, of course, are assumed constant. If, for example, some repairs were particularly complicated or required special skills (e.g., plumbing or electrical wiring), the likelihood of the use of a contractor rises.

6. The idea of a household producing housing services for itself is discussed more fully in Appendix G of Ozanne and Struyk (1976).

7. Longer distance moves are more often motivated by economic opportunity.

8. For a review see Quigley and Weinberg (1977).

9. Hanushek and Quigley (1978) use a formulation of this type in analyzing the moving behavior of renters in the Housing Allowance Demand Experiment.

10. Stated alternatively, the higher the transaction costs of moving, the longer the expected stay in a unit, and the more we can expect post move consumption patterns to reflect future events, such as increases in household size.

11. For this reason, a variety of alternatives will be tested, as discussed in Chapter 5.

12. It might be noted that the lagged value of the dependent variable will only appear as an independent variable in the model for repair and investment activity. There is no reason to expect similar habit formation in the other types of housing adjustments under consideration, namely, room use changes, taking in boarders, or making modifications to the unit.

13. Struyk (1982).

14. This summary appears in Struyk and Zais (1982), pp. 10-11.

15. In 1979 the Department of Housing and Urban Development fielded a supplement to the Annual Housing Survey in Houston as the first step in developing a longitudinal database on the housing of the elderly. The overall study, described in Newman (1979), was aborted; but the Houston data which does contain a battery of questions on room use change does exist. Ms. Newman is currently analyzing these data.

16. Room rental is distinguished from renting out a separate unit within the dwelling unit, for example, a basement apartment. While room rentals sometimes involve a rather separate space, such as a bedroom-bath combination in an attic or basement, they often are simply renting an extra bedroom with some of the home's main rooms shared in common by the family and boarder.

17. See Select Committee on Aging (1982); Hare (1980); Murray (1979).

18. Howe et al. (1984) review results and characteristics of several "home matching" programs involving the elderly.

19. See Helbers (1978) and Jacobs (1982) for further discussion and estimates.

20. U.S. Bureau of the Census, Survey of Residential Repairs and Alterations, Series C-50.

21. The pioneering study of in-place adjustment was completed by Mendelsohn (1977) who estimated a model for the demand for home improvements using cross-sectional data collected by the Bureau of the Census. The data lacked such variables as the size and initial condition of the unit, the stock of housing in the neighborhood, the health status of family members, the sex of the household head, and the household composition in general. Nevertheless, the results point to significant differences between elderly and nonelderly households. The elderly appear to make improvements significantly less often and they were much more likely to hire outside labor.

Helbers (1979), like Mendelsohn before him, used cross-sectional data and estimated independently the decision to make a repair to the unit and the amount to be spent. Using data on elderly homeowners in two midwestern cities, he took the additional step of disaggregating by household type (age, marital status, sex of head). His results amplify and are consistent with those of Mendelsohn. He did find differences between the two cities, which suggests that market characteristics such as the housing stock have important impact on in-place adjustment behavior.

22. For more on these issues see Moon (1977).

23. For some indicative figures on this point see Schwartz et al. (1984), Table 2.

24. As discussed below even though those living alone on average need less assistance, at the same time they receive more formal help, reflecting the lack of informal caregivers.

25. The source for these figures is Struyk (1982), Table 1.

26. It is not possible to compare these figures with the ones cited above, since these are households and the earlier ones were for individuals, and are designed to capture different types of needs.

27. This review generally cites only that literature directly used; readers may wish to consult these articles for a large number of further references.

28. The definition is given in the notes to Table 2.4.

29. For more on the determinants of the use of informal long-term care assistance see Branch and Jette (1983).

30. The definition of "unmarried" is not strictly comparable with the definition of "alone" used by other researchers. Also, see Verbrugge (1979), Greenberg and Ginn (1979), and Brody et al. (1978). On the other hand, Wolf (1983) does not find that the presence of a disability has a significant effect on the choice of living arrangements of the elderly.

31. It may be important to note that in this study the results were based on measures which excluded the spouse from the analyses so that informal social supports of the married person would be comparable to the widowed and the extent of support was estimated regardless of marital status.

32. For national estimates computed somewhat differently see Soldo (1982).

33. The sample on which this analysis relies is for part of New York State; we were not able to find comparable tabulations of national data which included all of the sources of services individually identified.

34. This is not to imply that all persons who need services receive them. Many of those who do not receive them are institutionalized.

35. For more on service utilization see, for example, Goodman (1984) and Johnson and Catalano (1983).

36. Sangl (1983), Horowitz et al. (1983), Reece et al. (1983).

37. One could argue to the contrary, for example, that poor conditions would make marketing the unit to potential boarders more difficult. This factor seems small compared to others determining the presence of boarders and for this reason is excluded.

38. For more on recent trends in the housing circumstances of the elderly, see Struyk and Turner (1984).

39. Department of Energy (1980), Table 1B.

40. For a thorough presentation of the empirical results for 39 metropolitan areas, see Follain and Malpezzi (1980).

41. Struyk-Soldo (1980), Chapter 6.

Chapter 3

The Data

The analysis in the next two chapters is based on a sample of 364 households who live in seven large central cities in the United States. These data were gathered as part of this project and track the surveyed households for a period of 57 months—an extensive period over which in-place housing adjustments were observed. The sample includes 177 households headed by an elderly person (defined as someone 60 years of age or older at the time of the second survey wave) and 187 households headed by a nonelderly person. The sample of the nonelderly was included to provide a base against which to compare the housing adjustments made by the elderly. This should enable us to identify those aspects which really distinguish such changes made by the elderly.

This chapter consists of three parts, all of which deal with the data acquired for this analysis. In the first part the complex program of data assembly is outlined, and the sample sizes in each of the seven sites at the end of the survey activity given. The second part outlines the content of the principal survey—the survey of households—which was fielded five times over the course of the project. The final part comments on the degree to which the resulting sample of households can be considered to be representative of all households residing in urban areas.

SURVEY DESIGN AND SAMPLE SIZES

The key to understanding the structure of the data collection is that the original data collection associated with this project extended a two-panel longitudinal household survey undertaken for another research project: the Community Development Strategies Evaluation (CDSE), which was sponsored by the Department of Housing and Urban Development, which funds the Community Development Block Grant program. Hence, this discussion begins by looking at the original survey activity associated with the CDSE. Then we describe the additional data collection of this project. A final section provides sample sizes available for analysis.

The Original Surveys and Sample

The 1974 Housing and Community Development Act integrated seven existing categorical programs administered by the Department of Housing and Urban Development (HUD) into a single Community Development Block Grant (CDBG). The 1974 Act embodies a broad philosophical shift away from direct federal control, within a set of broadly defined purposes specified in the law. The CDSE study is designed to determine how particular CDBG-funded activities (e.g., housing rehabilitation, urban redevelopment, public service provision), alone or in combination, influence the level and types of program achievements as well as the distribution of the benefits and costs to the population.

The CDSE was an ambitious attempt to perform an evaluation of the impact of the CDBG program in large cities. The project was initiated in 1978, and the main survey activity spanned the period from winter of 1979 to the first quarter of 1981. Since the effects of different types of community development strategies and city environments were of interest, HUD ultimately decided to concentrate the resources available for the study on neighborhoods in nine large (over 100,000 population) central cities. Selected for diversity in their community development activities, variation in regional location and size, and because they all had reasonably good data on their community development activities, these cities were: St. Paul, Wichita, Corpus Christi, Memphis, New Haven, Denver, Pittsburgh, San Francisco, Birmingham.

The total of 20 neighborhoods within these cities selected for intensive analysis in the CDSE are central to the data collection and analysis undertaken in this study. In particular, the variance in neighborhood investment climate is likely to be important in explaining the extent of in-place housing adjustments. The strategy used in the CDSE for selecting candidate neighborhoods balanced the following criteria:

— diversity in neighborhood context (housing stock, tenure, household income, ethnic composition, and family structure);
— diversity in community development activities in neighborhoods, i.e., housing rehabilitation, public facilities and infrastructure, redevelopment, and combinations of these activities;
— inclusion in the sample of at least two neighborhoods from each of the nine sample cities;
— use of a sampling ratio for households which is sufficient in each of the neighborhoods to permit inference to be possible for those spatial units;
— avoidance of straddling the boundaries of locally perceived "natural" (or ecological) neighborhoods; and
— use of contiguous "census blocks" to define neighborhoods to permit comparison with the 1970 and possibly 1980 census data.

Overall, the objective in neighborhood selection was to insure enough variance in neighborhood conditions and community development "treatments" to permit analysis of the importance of these effects.[1] The 20 neighborhoods selected each contain approximately sample 100 households in 25 contiguous blocks. The diversity of the neighborhoods is depicted in Table 3.1. As indicated by 1970 census tract statistics, some of the neighborhoods had moderate household income, others can be judged to be "low income." Twelve of the neighborhoods have a higher minority representation including black, Hispanic, and Oriental populations. A number of neighborhoods had a high representation of families with children, as opposed to single young adults or elderly single people. Owner-occupancy prevails in five of the neighborhoods. In general, each major demographic variable shows a wide degree of variation.[2]

Since a substantial and varied data collection program to support longitudinal analyses of benefits and program impacts was required, 11 different types of surveys were conducted in the study.

TABLE 3.1

DEMOGRAPHIC CHARACTERISTICS OF NEIGHBORHOODS, ORIGINAL CASE STUDY

CITY/ NEIGHBORHOOD	RACE			MEDIAN INCOME $	TENURE		HOUSEHOLD COMPOSITION				
					% Single-Family, Owner Occupant	% Multiple-Family, Owner Occupant	Single		Couples		Other
	% White	% Black	% Other				With Children	Without Children	With Children	Without Children	
St. Paul											
St. Anthony/Midway	94.3	0.9	4.7	12,343	29.2	5.7	8.4	40.4	18.9	21.7	10.4
Westside	77.6	.9	21.3	11,526	45.2	4.8	17.3	31.2	30.7	15.4	4.8
Memphis											
Binghampton	1.0	98.9	0.0	7,600	35.1	0.0	23.7	23.7	25.7	19.6	7.2
Parkway/Lauderdale	0.0	98.9	1.0	5,882	38.7	2.2	34.7	34.7	14.1	10.9	5.4
Pittsburgh											
Beltzhoover	18.4	81.5	0.0	11,971	65.2	3.3	17.3	20.6	11.3	9.9	6.5
Manchester	19.2	79.4	1.2	10,083	31.6	10.1	17.7	41.7	17.7	17.6	5.1
Wichita											
McAdams	4.3	95.6	0.0	6,803	43.8	2.1	19.7	40.6	9.3	20.8	9.4
Plainview	85.7	10.9	3.2	9,998	30.9	6.4	15.9	25.3	33.0	22.3	3.2

New Haven											
Dwight	60.2	37.3	2.5	10,924	1.2	4.7	9.4	61.2	4.6	13.0	11.8
Fair Haven	77.6	4.2	18.0	9,995	4.1	33.0	21.6	26.6	23.7	24.7	3.1
Newhallville	7.4	91.3	1.2	11,062	24.4	15.9	21.9	13.3	32.9	19.4	13.4
San Francisco											
Alamo Square	48.1	43.0	8.8	14,375	4.9	4.9	9.8	49.3	9.8	8.6	22.2
Bernal Heights	71.4	14.7	2.3	16,422	44.0	11.9	14.2	30.8	11.8	25.0	17.9
Inner Mission	24.0	2.4	73.4	11,438	13.6	9.1	28.7	19.3	31.0	12.6	8.0
Corpus Christi											
Census Tract 9	1.8	0.9	87.1	8,576	59.4	1.9	12.2	24.5	43.3	16.0	3.8
Census Tract 16	1.8	11.3	86.7	9,062	74.1	0.0	17.5	16.5	41.6	18.6	5.6
Denver											
Highland Park	53.8	0.0	46.2	12,348	50.0	2.1	13.8	29.7	29.8	22.3	4.3
Whittier	8.0	81.8	10.2	8,246	32.7	2.0	35.3	26.1	18.1	9.0	10.9
Birmingham											
Wylam	87.7	11.3	0.0	11,168	74.8	17.8	9.3	27.0	27.1	29.0	7.5
N. Birmingham	16.8	83.1	0.0	10,186	65.7	2.8	20.5	18.6	35.4	17.6	7.4

We use data from four of these and based our survey instruments on their design, where applicable.

Additional Data Collection

Because this analysis is focused primarily on elderly homeowners living in single-family dwellings, before undertaking additional data collection in any of the nine cities, we examined the number of elderly and nonelderly homeowners in the sample for each city. For two cities — New Haven and San Francisco — we determined that the number of elderly homeowners was too small to warrant the expense of establishing field operations in the sites. Consequently, our field work extended the CDSE surveys in 14 neighborhoods in seven cities.

Table 3.2 summarizes the overall data collection activity. All surveys conducted after the first quarter of 1981 are post-CDSE. The chart shows that three additional waves of household surveys were conducted, for a total of five spanning a period of approximately 57 months. The household survey was not, however, conducted at the same time interval throughout the period: about 18 months separated waves 1 and 2, and waves 2 and 3; but only 12 months separated each of the last three waves. A shorter time period was used for the post-CDSE waves because of our concern about recall problems over a period longer than a year, especially for the elderly.[3]

We were particularly concerned about potential recall problems for repairs, maintenance, and modest improvements to the home. The Census Bureau in its survey of such activities uses a quarterly panel design, in which households remain in the surveyed group for several quarters, to overcome problems of underestimation found when an annual reporting period was used.[4] To minimize the underreporting we used a supplemental telephone survey at four month intervals between the household surveys, beginning the fourth month after the third household survey.[5] As a result of these procedures, we have substantially greater confidence in the data for the last two years of the observation period on repairs and improvements than for the earlier 33 months.

As indicated in Table 3.2, we have also made use of data gath-

TABLE 3.2

DATA COLLECTION SCHEDULE[a]

Time		dwelling unit inspection inspection	windshield survey	household survey	dwelling repairs and investment survey
1979	Q4	X	X	X	X[b]
1981	Q1			X	X[b]
1982	Q3			X	X[b]
	Q4				X
1983	Q1				X
	Q2				
	Q3			X	X[b]
	Q4				
1984	Q1				X
	Q2			X	X
	Q3				X[b]

a. "X" indicates date of fielding; in the case of the "independent" dwelling and repair surveys, indicates date of phone calls.
b. Asked as part of household survey.

63

ered in two "one-time" surveys conducted within the CDSE. The first is a highly-detailed, room-by-room, inspection of the dwelling done by professional appraisers. The data from this instrument give a very accurate depiction of the condition of the unit at the start of the observation period. The second instrument — the windshield survey — provides parallel information on the immediate area (the "block face") on which the dwelling is located. Information is included on land use, type and condition of residential structure, presence of nuisances, and similar attributes of the area.

Finally, two points should be noted about the procedures employed in constructing the files used in this analysis. First, all survey records regarding an individual household and its dwelling were linked, thus yielding a comprehensive database for each observation. This greatly facilitated analyses involving tracking changes in the household's status, e.g., economic position over time. Second, because the number of observations in each of the elderly and nonelderly household files is quite small, it was necessary to impute values where they were missing in the raw survey file for all of the variables used in the analysis. This turned out to be an extensive task, but one which was absolutely essential for performing the analysis reported in the next two chapters.[6]

Terminal Sample Sizes

The final sample sizes, disaggregated by age of household head and site, are shown in Table 3.3. As shown in the table, end-of-period samples of households headed by an elderly person range from 14 in Denver to 29 in Wichita and Birmingham. These very

TABLE 3.3

FINAL SAMPLE SIZES BY CITY AND AGE
OF HOUSEHOLD HEAD
(number of households)

City	Non-elderly	Elderly	Total
St. Paul	22	15	37
Memphis	22	26	48
Pittsburgh	29	23	52
Wichita	11	29	40
Corpus Christi	46	41	87
Denver	11	14	25
Birmingham	46	29	75

small individual site samples unfortunately preclude any site-specific analysis.

From wave 3 to wave 5 of the household survey, the sample experienced only moderate attrition – about 6% per year. This is quite low considering that any household who moved away was lost from the sample as well as those refusing to participate in the surveys. Response burden was quite heavy for these households, as they were asked to answer questions on seven different occasions beginning with the third household survey and this was after three previous survey encounters.[7] Even so the great majority of attrition was due to households relocating.

An attribute of considerable importance is the age distribution of the heads of households. Table 3.4 presents percentage distributions for nonelderly and elderly headed households for the sample of households surviving until the end of the observation period. Ages are as of the second household survey wave. The sample of nonelderly households is quite concentrated in the middle-aged

TABLE 3.4

AGE DISTRIBUTION OF HEADS OF HOUSEHOLDS IN THE
SAMPLES OF NON-ELDERLY AND ELDERLY HOUSEHOLDS

Age of Household Head	Percent in Class
Nonelderly head	
21-25	2
26-30	7
31-35	8
36-40	12
41-45	12
46-50	13
51-55	20
56-60	25
Elderly head	
61-65	27
66-70	23
71-75	23
76-80	14
81-85	5
85+	8

group: 45% are between ages 51 and 60, and 58% are between 46 and 60. Likewise, most of the elderly households (73%) are within 15 years of the age 60 dividing line. The large share of the nonelderly population which is very near to age 60 at only the second survey wave implies that some of the contrasts between the nonelderly and elderly populations will not be as sharp as they would be if the nonelderly group were somewhat younger. Unfortunately, the beginning sample sizes were not great enough to permit us to sharpen the contrasts by dividing the sample households into three groups of young, middle-aged, and elderly for the analysis.

INSTRUMENT CONTENT

The household survey fielded in waves 3-5 and the corresponding telephone survey of dwelling repairs and improvements were designed to obtain information on the types of housing adjustments and causal factors discussed in the last chapter. Consequently, it is not surprising that Table 3.5, which lists the subject areas covered by the various surveys, should resemble the list of variables from that chapter.

The table shows that three of the four instruments covered only a single topic area. The principal instrument was clearly the household survey, in terms of the number of different areas covered. The entries in the column for the household survey indicate in which survey waves a subject area was covered. There was a major shift in coverage at the third wave, the point at which the CDSE sample was taken over for further study in this project. It is important to note that wherever possible the same questions were continued on the survey throughout all five waves.[8] This was particularly the case for information on living arrangements, the household's economic position, and a short set of questions on the condition of the dwelling unit. The additional areas included beginning in the third wave covered additional types of housing adjustments, the presence and extent of activity limitations by household members, the degree of aid these persons received from various sources, and the type and degree of social interaction outside of the home experienced by the head or spouse.[9]

It should also be noted that beginning with the third wave the date

TABLE 3.5

SUMMARY OF SUBJECT AREAS COVERED IN DIFFERENT SURVEYS

Subject Area	dwelling unit inspection[a]	windshield survey[a]	household survey[b]	dwelling repair & investment survey[a]
1. Housing adjustments				
- room use changes			3-5	
- dwelling modifications			3-5	
- presence of boarders			1-5	
- repairs & investment in dwelling			1-3	X
2. Economic position				
- income, assets, debts			1-5	
- housing expenditures			1-5	
3. Living arrangements			1-5	
4. Social interaction/support			3-5	
5. Supportive services			3-5	
6. Activity limitations			3-5	
7. Dwelling condition	X		1-5	
8. Neighborhood conditions		X		
9. Plans to move			1-5	

a. "X" indicates that area was covered in the survey.
b. Numbers indicate the survey waves in which the area was included.

at which various important events occurred was included. In the third wave, for example, if the respondent reported an activity limitation, he was asked when the limitation had first occurred. In subsequent waves the respondent would have been asked about the month since the last interview when a limitation, if reported, had begun. Such monthly "dates" were recorded for most types of housing adjustments, income changes, and changes in living arrangements, activity limitations, support services and social interaction. These data lay the foundation for a more precise analysis of the ordering in time of housing adjustments and the causes for them.

From the foregoing description it is clear that a very large data set has been assembled for the 364 households included in our sample. The analysis variables constructed alone number around 1,300 for each observation. Especially important, however, is the fact that this single data set contains variables from all domains of conceptual interest.

REPRESENTATIVENESS

Given the purpose for which the original sample was drawn and the fact that households were drawn from particular neighborhoods within a small number of cities, one does not anticipate that the households included in this analysis will be representative of all of those in urban areas in this country. Nevertheless, it is useful to know the ways in which this sample differs from the population of households, so that tabulations done based on them can be appropriately interpreted.[10] Hence, this section briefly summarizes the two tests conducted, which are described more fully in Appendix A.

The first test is for differences between several key attributes of the households sampled for this study versus those sampled from the central cities of metropolitan areas in the Current Population Survey. The tabulations show that the households in this study are on average significantly older and poorer than those in central cities generally, although the two groups are similarly distributed among different household types.

The second test compares the attributes of the neighborhoods from which the sample employed in this study are drawn with neighborhoods in central cities generally. All attributes considered were taken from 1980 census tract data. Of six attributes considered, the two groups of places were found to differ in terms of racial composition and the share of families headed by a woman, with our sample neighborhoods having a higher proportion of minorities and female headed households. They were similar in terms of the percentage of elderly present, and the percentage of dwellings which were owner-occupied, lacked complete plumbing, and were vacant.

On the basis of these simple comparisons, one would have to consider the sample used here as nonrepresentative in important dimensions. The results presented in the next two chapters, which are based on data that have *not* been weighted to adjust for these differences, should be treated accordingly.

NOTES

1. For further discussion, see Ginsberg et al. (1980) and the University of Pennsylvania (1980).

2. Field reconnaissance for the original study indicated that citizen participation was relatively high in nine of the areas and that six of the neighborhoods could be classified as located in the core of their cities, eight were in an intermediate location, and six were peripheral to the core. Systematic differences in the type and magnitude of community development assistance are also evident. Five neighborhoods were affected principally by infrastructure investments alone without significant housing rehabilitation. Rehabilitation without major investments in public facilities occurred in five other neighborhoods. Substantial investment in both housing rehabilitation and public facilities occurred in seven neighborhoods. Three areas had some prior redevelopment experience in addition to housing rehabilitation and infrastructure.

3. See Ridley et al. (1979).

4. Analysis of daily activity (time logs) suggest more activity of this type than even quarterly interviews; see Hill (1980).

5. The same "telephone survey instrument" was used at the time of the fourth and fifth household survey waves. A copy of this instrument is provided in a companion report documenting the analysis file, Katsura and Struyk (1985).

6. An overview of these procedures is given Appendix B.

7. We are not able to construct accurate attrition rates for the full sample period. This is the case because, when the files for the first two survey waves were transferred to us, some observations were missing that had not been indicated as nonrespondents by the survey firm (the National Opinion Research Corporation). These households may have been dropped because we had requested records from the University of Pennsylvania for only those households for which information

from all the surveys—including the dwelling unit inspection and windshield survey—was present. Attempts to sort these problems out were thwarted by the fact that the CDSE project was in its final stages and the people most knowledgeable about the data set had already departed.

Note that about a dozen additional cases were dropped because we had to impute a large number of values for missing data items. Our view was that the household record was becoming excessively synthetic because of these imputations.

8. We were very fortunate in having the National Opinion Research Center conduct all five household survey waves. In most cases the same interviewers were available for the entire project, providing important continuity in reporting and helping assure high continued participation rates by the sample households.

9. The household survey used in the third survey wave and in the telephone dwelling repair and improvement instruments are reproduced in Katsura and Struyk (1985). Further discussion of the reason for including specific questions in the instrument is provided in Struyk (1982).

10. In contrast, the results of the multivariate analysis presented in Chapter 5 should not suffer from this problem. For an explanation for this result, see Dumochel and Duncan (1977).

Chapter 4

Incidence and Dynamics

In this chapter we present data on the incidence of housing adjustments made without households relocating and of changes in demographic, health, and financial factors that may affect these adjustments. The primary focus, however, is on the patterns of change over the observation period: is the dominant pattern among households having boarders present to have one in the home throughout the period or is their presence episodic? Do households consistently make several repairs to their units or does this vary sharply from year-to-year? Similar questions are asked about changes in factors affecting adjustments: is the degree of social support provided by children no longer living at home at about the same level year after year? Do people report the same degree of activity and mobility limitations in successive interviews or do their perceptions of their status change? How variable is the amount of informal and paid support services received by households who claim that they need such services? How violently does a family's economic position change from year-to-year?

Answering the type of question just posed for a sample of households drawn from different parts of the country will provide more information than has been available to date on the dynamics of elderly housing adjustments. It will also provide a more complete picture of the overall degree of change in the lives of the elderly living in their own homes. Thus, these patterns are of substantial interest in their own right and understanding them is essential for interpreting the results of the multivariate analysis presented in the next chapter. Of course, the limitations of our sample, described in Chapter 3, should be kept in mind throughout.

A problem in presenting these data is to determine what degree of change over the observation period constitutes a "substantial or significant" degree of change. The problem arises because our data set permits us to do the initial exploration of many of these patterns. We use two bases for comparison. First, since our primary interest is on households headed by an elderly person, we use the data for the parallel panel of nonelderly households as a reference point for many of the patterns. Second, it is often possible to contrast the extent of change among variables measuring the same phenomena, such as activity limitations or economic circumstances. These techniques permit us to say a good deal about the patterns observed, but they nevertheless leave us without any absolute measures of "significant rates of change."

As an aid in examining the patterns of change, we have developed a simple scheme for classifying each variable. As noted in the last chapter, we have five observations over time for each household for many of the analysis variables and three observations for most of the rest. For example, we have five observations on whether the head of the household is female. One can depict schematically the case in which a household has a female head at the start of the period but a male head in all successive waves as XOOOO; or the case in which there is a one-time shift from female to male at wave three as XXOOO. Finally, a more dynamic case might be OOXOX. We constructed summaries like these for all of the variables employed in the analysis. In addition, we developed the following classification scheme to summarize the large number of possible patterns of Xs and Os:

> *stable* — no change in the household over time; this would include both the XXXXX and OOOOO patterns.

> *one-time change* — there is a single change that is sustained over the balance of the period; this would include OOXXX, for example.

> *dynamic* — there is more than one change over the period; examples of such patterns include XOXOX, XOOOX, and OXXXO.

We make one further distinction within the stable group by distinguishing between those households who always have some attribute and those that never have it. So for example, in studying repair activity we distinguish among households classified as stable between those who never made a repair to the interior of their home and those that made such a repair in every period.

While this classification scheme provides a powerful tool for interpreting the patterns of change, it is limited in several ways. First, the classifications themselves are naturally very sensitive to reporting error or to misclassification that might have been introduced in imputing missing values.[1] A single incorrect response could shift an observation from a stable to dynamic classification, e.g., XXXXX vs. XOXXX. Second, changes at the beginning and end of the observation period may be, respectively, the end or start of a more complex set of adjustments. Hence, this scheme can understate the actual amount of change ongoing. For example, we would classify the pattern XXXXO as a one-time change; if we had observed it for a single year more, however, it might have been classified as dynamic, i.e., XXXOX.

This brings us to another difficulty: comparison of patterns for different numbers of observations. Depending on the variable, we have from three to six observations for it. Clearly the chances of a "stable" pattern diminish as the number of observations rises (either because the time covered increases and there are more chances for real change or because there are more opportunities for reporting errors); and the chances for a "dynamic" pattern correspondingly increase. Additionally, the smaller the number of observations the higher the likelihood of "incomplete patterns" in which one only observes the end or start of a more complex set of changes. For example, we might observe OXX when the full five observation pattern might be XXOXX; in the former case the variable would have been categorized as a one-time change, in the latter as dynamic.

A further problem in interpreting the degree of change between successive survey waves is that the time period between waves varies significantly. As discussed in the last chapter, the time between household survey waves 1-2 and 2-3 is about 18 months, while that between 3-4 and 4-5 is a year. Naturally one expects more change over the longer periods. Analytically there is little that can be done to make the kind of computations measuring change employed here more comparable when they are based on differing numbers of observations or have differing time periods between observations. Nevertheless, we believe these measures provide a very useful summary measure and we employ them often.

The balance of this chapter presents the information we have developed on the incidence of various events and their dynamics. It begins with data on the housing adjustments made over the observation period and proceeds on a domain-by-domain basis to cover dwelling conditions, living arrangements and other demographics, social interaction and support, the need for and receipt of supportive services, and the household's economic position. Most of the following data are simple tabulations presented separately for nonelderly headed and elderly headed households. While a few cross-tabulations are included, the small size of the samples precludes doing much analysis of this type.

HOUSING ADJUSTMENTS

We look first at housing adjustments other than repairs and improvements to the dwelling; these include taking in roomers or boarders, making modifications to the dwelling to permit someone with a disability to use it more fully, and changing the use of rooms in the dwelling. A principal finding about these adjustments is their low incidence of occurrence. Table 4.1 presents information on such adjustments during the period covered by survey waves 3-5 (W3-W5).²

Boarders are extremely rare among nonelderly headed households, with only about 1% of these households renting out a room. Even among the elderly, however, only as many as 3% take in a boarder in any year. Table 4.2 provides information on the pattern of changes over the three survey waves in several types of housing adjustments, following the scheme described earlier. The second panel of the data in the table is for roomers and boarders. It shows for the elderly, for example, that 95% had no roomers over the period, none had a roomer throughout the period and in general the pattern of the presence of a roomer was quite unstable. This finding is consistent with those from studies using shorter observation periods and suggests the difficulties of constructing a satisfactory house sharing arrangement.

Although the number of roomers in homes owned by the elderly is very small, one may obtain some rough idea of the living arrangements from the answers to several additional questions included in the surveys on this point. According to these data, only about 20% of the boarders provided help around the house. In addition, while the person in the home had some contact with the boarder in three out of four cases, "social contact" — in the sense of sharing meals or evenings together — was very rare. Thus, at least in the handful of cases covered in this survey, the elderly would obtain little social support or assistance from renting out a room. This may in part explain the high turnover in roomers.

We turn now to *modifications made to the dwelling* to enhance its compatibility with one or more family members with activity limitations. The figures in Table 4.1 show moderate levels of such modifications being made. It is important to note that the question asked at W3 was about all modifications *installed by the household up to that time*; the parallel questions in W4 and W5 were about modifications installed in the last year. Up to the time of the W3 survey, the average home occupied by a nonelderly headed family had .06 modifications and the average home occupied by the elderly had .21 modifications. After allowing for multiple modifications to some homes, 19% of homes occupied by elderly headed households and 4% of those occupied by the nonelderly had at least one modification. Thereafter, both groups of households annually made modifications equivalent to an average of about .05 average changes per unit. Overall this is a sharply higher extent of modifications than one would have expected based on prior studies.

Among the modifications made, by far the most common are those we have classified as moderate — installation of extra handrails and grab bars; push bars; flashing lights; and changing sink, faucets, and cabinets to be easier for the impaired person to use. This pattern holds for nonelderly headed households as well as the elderly.

The third panel of Table 4.2 shows the pattern of implementing

TABLE 4.1

INCIDENCE OF CHANGES IN DWELLING USAGE, WAVES 3-5
(percents)

	Non-elderly Headed			Elderly Headed		
	W3	W4	W5	W3	W4	W5
Boarders present						
Number of boarders: 1	1	-	1	3	2	1
2+	1	-	1	2	2	1
	-	-	-	1	-	-
Dwelling modifications:[a]						
Total no. of modifications[b]	.06	.05	.04	.21	.04	.09
No. of extensive modifications[b]	-	-	.01	.01	.01	.01
No. of moderate[c]	.04	.02	.02	.16	.01	.05
No. of small[d]	.01	.02	.01	.02	-	-
Room use changes, since last interview:						
Any changes? (percent)	6	4	2	5	3	2
Of those with changes, no. of changes of each type						
– new bathroom	.08	-	-	-	-	-
– new bedroom	.17	.25	.75	.33	.20	.25
– other	.92	.75	.25	.67	.80	.75

a. In wave 3 the question concerned all modifications made to that time; question in subsequent waves asked about changes made since the last interview.

b. Includes ramps, elevators, and modifying a bathroom for wheelchair use.

c. Includes extra handrails and grab bars, extra wide doors, push bars, flashing lights, and modifications of sinks, faucets, or cabinets.

d. Includes door handles, braille labels, special wall sockets, and specially equipped telephones.

TABLE 4.2

PATTERNS OF HOUSING ADJUSTMENT OVER TIME
(percents)

	Non-elderly Headed Households					Elderly Headed Households				
	stable		total	one-time shift	dynamic	stable		total	one-time shift	dynamic
	high	low				high	low			
Annual Repairs (5 obs.):										
Any repairs done?	54	1	55	18	27	35	–	35	22	43
Any interior repairs?	35	1	36	20	44	19	2	21	26	53
Any exterior repairs?	10	7	17	25	58	7	4	11	30	59
Any moderate repairs?	16	2	18	31	51	8	4	12	27	61
Any major repairs?	1	46	47	14	39	–	56	56	16	28
Boarder (5 obs.):										
Boarder present	1	97	98	1	1	–	95	95	2	3
Unit modifications (3 obs.):										
Any modification in period	1	93	94	3	3	1	74	75	24	1
Type of mod.: extensive	–	99	99	1	–	–	97	97	2	1
moderate	–	95	95	3	2	–	80	80	19	1
small	1	97	98	1	1	–	98	98	2	–
Room changes (3 obs.):										
Any room change	–	88	88	9	3	1	91	92	6	2
Memorandum item:										
Any boarder present over the period	3					5				

modifications over the period. Among both the elderly and nonelderly headed households about 1% reported modifying their unit in each of the three periods (see the results for "any modifications in period"). Even among the elderly, however, a substantial majority (74%) undertook no modifications. Among the balance of households who made some modification over the period, only 2 of the 25% reported making a modification in more than one year.

The number of households making *changes in the use of rooms* over a one year period is also fairly low, but perhaps higher than one might have imagined. Among both nonelderly and elderly headed households about 5% make such a change annually (Table 4.1). Among the changes made the most common is to a purpose other than a bedroom or bathroom. In fact, the dominant pattern is from a bedroom to a special purpose room, such as a sewing room, work room, or office. Still about one-third of the new room uses are bedrooms. As one might imagine, changing the use of rooms does not occur often within the same house (Table 4.2). There are only two cases of the same household making more than one such change over the period.[3]

The general picture that emerges of these three types of housing adjustments is that they are highly discrete changes which households undertake quite rarely. The low average incidence combined with the fact that those households undertaking them only themselves make a single change, i.e., do not repeat the change for several years, suggests that the causal modeling of the determinants of these events may be difficult.

The final housing adjustment to be discussed are *repairs and improvements* made to the dwelling unit. This discussion is closely related to changes in dwelling condition over time presented in the next section, since the hypothesis is that those households undertaking little dwelling upkeep will find their units deteriorating. At this point we examine the extent of repairs and improvement activity.

Table 4.3 shows the mean values for the total number of activities undertaken and their cost for the periods covered by all five survey waves separately for households headed by nonelderly and elderly persons, respectively. Some caution is in order in looking at these figures as they cover differing periods of time and, except for the last two waves, different seasons of the year. Even so, three

TABLE 4.3

MEAN NUMBER AND TOTAL COST OF REPAIRS AND IMPROVEMENTS
FOR EACH SURVEY WAVE

	Age of Head of Household			
	Non-elderly		Elderly	
Survey Wave	Repairs	Cost	Repairs	Cost
1a	3.46	$ 1,864	2.43	$ 1,160
2b	3.36	1,991	2.27	1,130
3b	2.70	1,224	1.90	1,036
4a	3.77	765	2.81	669
5a	4.27	1,167	2.81	718

a. Covers one-year period.
b. Covers approximately 18 month period.

patterns stand out. The first is the high average level of expenditures on repairs and improvements, compared to values reported in surveys conducted by the Bureau of the Census.[4] Additionally, the small average number of repairs implies a very high average cost for the repairs and improvements reported—on the order of $200. The second point is the volatility of the mean values of repairs and improvements over time. From period-to-period the shifts are as large as several hundred dollars; since some of these occur among the last three waves, they cannot be attributed solely to differing reporting periods. This point is reinforced by an examination of the movements of the sample households among five groups (no repairs reported and four quartiles for those reporting repairs) between survey waves (see Table C.3, p.184). Only about one-fourth of the households remain in the same group between any pair of surveys and about one-third of them move more than one group, e.g., from no repairs to the third quartile. Finally, both the values of expenditures on and the number of repairs and improvements reported is consistently larger for nonelderly households than for the elderly.

In Chapter 3 we noted that during the last two years of the survey period we had gathered data on repairs and improvements thrice yearly to improve the accuracy of the information obtained. Some summary statistics based on these four-month observations are presented in Table 4.4. The column heads show the survey wave number and the season of the year (Summer or Winter) to help orient the

TABLE 4.4

REPAIR ACTIVITY IN FOUR MONTH PERIODS IN LAST TWO SURVEY YEARS

	Non-elderly Headed Households						Elderly Headed Households					
For all respondents:	1/s[a]	2/w	3/s	4/w	5/w	6/s	1/s	2/w	3/s	4/w	5/w	6/s
Any repairs done?	.64	.56	.70	.59	.58	.70	.48	.40	.65	.52	.41	.60
Total no. of repairs	1.26	1.06	1.54	1.30	1.30	1.68	.87	.65	1.31	.86	.74	1.21
Total cost of repairs ($)	266	217	300	399	223	546	207	165	302	176	153	390
Total interior repairs	.99	.79	1.05	1.01	.89	1.12	.59	.48	.85	.66	.48	.82
Total exterior repairs	.24	.21	.43	.25	.40	.50	.27	.16	.42	.20	.25	.35
Total moderate repairs[b]	.39	.30	.48	.35	.38	.59	.28	.25	.56	.26	.26	.47
Total major repairs[c]	.05	.04	.06	.06	.04	.09	.04	.03	.03	.03	.02	.06
Any renovations?[d]	.03	.04	.05	.04	.01	.05	.01	.01	.03	-	.01	.03
For those with any repairs:												
Share of work done by[e]												
- head or spouse	.48	.40	.61	.55	.63	.55	.35	.33	.26	.22	.30	.25
- other household members or relatives	.06	.06	.04	.08	.07	.09	.05	.08	.24	.15	.19	.08
- friends, neighbors	.06	.04	.04	.05	.06	.04	.18	.09	.16	.15	.15	.16
Mean value of repairs ($)	203	223	247	270	173	415	205	263	245	246	199	303

a. "s" means that the period covered included mostly good (Summer) building weather; "w" means it contained mostly Winter weather.

b. Those costing $100-$1,000.

c. Those costing over $1,000.

d. Room remodeling or additions to a house.

e. Work done by persons other than contractors and without payment.

reader to the level of activity ongoing. The lower level of exterior repairs in winter months is a consistent pattern for both household groups.

A number of clear differences between households headed by a nonelderly person and those with an elderly head are evident. More of the nonelderly in every period make repairs or improvements and they undertake a larger number on average as well. Likewise, average total expenditures are consistently higher, as noted above. On the other hand, for those undertaking these actions, the mean value of repairs is about the same for the two groups (see the last row of the table). There are two types of repairs and improvements for which the difference in the percentage of households undertaking them is much closer between the nonelderly and the elderly than for the others. These are exterior repairs and major improvements. Intuitively, the need for exterior repairs in order to preserve the structural integrity of the unit is a powerful force in causing such repairs to be made. The similarity in the levels of major improvements (both those labeled in the table as major repairs and as "any major renovation"), on the other hand, is more difficult to surmise, although major changes associated with dwelling modifications among the elderly is certainly reasonable. A seemingly high share — around 3% — of both the nonelderly and elderly report major repairs or major renovations each period, which helps account for the high average repair values in Table 4.3.[5]

Interesting but expected differences are also evident in the patterns of who actually does the work involved in the repair or improvement. Four categories are distinguished: head or spouse; other household member or relative not living there; friend or neighbor; and contractors. The last group is not shown in the table. While in households headed by a nonelderly person a little over half of all repairs are done by the head or spouse, in elderly households the figure is about 30%. By contrast, others in the household, friends, and neighbors provide little help to the nonelderly (about 10-12% of repairs are done by them), but account for about 25% of the repairs done to units occupied by the elderly. Contractors are quite important to both groups.

The first panel of Table 4.2 shows the consistency over time with which households undertake different kinds of repair activities. In every category the nonelderly are more likely to make repairs year after year than their elderly counterparts (as shown by the figures for "stable-high"). Still 35% of the elderly reported repairs for five consecutive years. On the other hand, 43% of the elderly were classified in the "dynamic" groups, indicating repair actions to be an "on again-off again" thing, compared with only 27% of the nonelderly. An important point is that over the period there were very few elderly households who did not at some time undertake all of the categories of repairs except major repairs (see the "stable-low" column). Thus, there is little evidence of a cohort of older homeowners simply ceasing to maintain their homes because of lack of money, know-how, or other reasons.

We have done further analysis of the extent of activity undertaken each year using both the total cost of repairs and improvements and the total number of repairs and improvements made as the measures. For each year each household was placed into one of five groups for each of these two measures: no activity, and those with some activity were classified into quartiles based on the extent of their expenditures or count of actions. We then cross-tabulated the results for succeeding years, thereby constructing a five by five matrix that revealed changes in position. An examination of these cross-tabulations shows a great deal of shifting of households among the various positions; at the same time quite a few households repeated their same position in succeeding years.[6]

These findings combined with the other patterns of repair and improvement activity reviewed earlier point to a general pattern of discrete decisions to undertake many such activities. While many households do make some repairs or improvements each year, the type of actions, their cost, and their number vary sharply over time. This broad finding applies to both groups of households examined, although the degree of continuity is clearly greater for households headed by a nonelderly person.

DWELLING ATTRIBUTES AND CONDITIONS

As indicated at several earlier points, prevention of housing deficiencies or remedying them after they have occurred are major motivations for dwelling repair and maintenance actions. In this section we first examine the quality profile of the dwelling units occupied by households included in our sample. Later we present some data on the configuration of these dwellings that could effect the need for dwelling modifications.

The top panel of Table 4.5 gives the incidence of various structural deficiencies at the start of the observation period. These measures were derived from the exceptionally detailed inventories of unit conditions that were conducted by trained observers at this time; these data were gathered only once over the study period. The incidence of any single problem is quite low with the exception of the absence or disrepair of stairs or essential railings and problems with the roof, either structural or surface. Combined, however,

TABLE 4.5

SELECTED DWELLING UNIT ATTRIBUTES
(percents)

	Age of Household Head	
Housing Problems	Non Elderly	Elderly
Significant problems with:[a]		
foundation	--	2
wall structure	2	7
wall surface	6	8
roof structure	14	14
roof surface	11	10
gutters and downspouts	3	2
stairs and railings	20	10
Overall rating by inspector:		
conditions immediately or potentially hazardous	5	12
quality: uninhabitable or low quality	18	20
Structural Configuration[b]		
Dwelling on one level[c]	67	72
Finished basement	31	30
Finished attic	16	15
For multi-story units only:		
o bedroom on 1st floor, no bathroom	8	12
o bath on 1st floor, no bedrooms	26	16
o bedroom and bath on 1st floor	34	30

a. At baseline.
b. At Wave 3 survey.
c. Excluding basement and attic.

these measures indicate that a substantial number of dwellings had a significant problem at the start of the observation period. To be precise, 23% of the unit occupied by households with a nonelderly head and 17% of those occupied by households with an elderly head had a structural problem.[7]

We can now obtain some idea of the persistence of dwelling deficiencies from the data in Table 4.6. These data are for a total of 10 problems with the unit about which the respondent was asked in either three or five survey waves. These are a rather different set of measures than those just discussed; they do not include structural problems, since the proper identification of these requires expert judgement. Rather the problems included here are generally manifestations of deficiencies. So, for example, a leaking roof may be indicative of structural or surface problems with the roof.

The top panel of Table 4.6 shows the patterns of persistence in five dwelling problems across all five survey waves. The majority of dwellings do not experience each of these problems over the entire period. The only problems experienced during the entire period by any household are leaking roofs and basements. The overall pattern is clearly one of households experiencing a problem and correcting it. It is important to note, however, that all five of the problems included in this set effect basic living conditions. Not dealing with a problem would definitely effect the quality of life adversely.

On the other hand, the problems listed in the lower part of the table all involve items that are less central to an adequate living environment. While we only have three observations for these items, the patterns still appear to be quite different from those just discussed. In particular, there is a high incidence of persistent problems for gutters being in poor condition. In addition, roughly 6 to 10% of the units exhibit each of the other problems as well year after year. Interestingly, the incidence of these problems for dwellings occupied by the elderly is essentially no different than that for those occupied by the nonelderly. Also, an examination of cross-tabulations of the presence of these problems with the total cost of repairs undertaken in a year reveals no systematic relationship.

The overall picture that emerges from these data is that the housing conditions of the elderly homeowners included in this sample

TABLE 4.6

CHANGES IN DWELLING CONDITIONS OVER TIME
(percents)

	Non-elderly Headed Households					Elderly Headed Households				
	stable			one-time			stable			one-time	
	good	poor	total	shift	dynamic	good	poor	total	shift	dynamic
Five Observations										
basement leaks	84	4	88	8	4	89	1	90	8	2
roof leaks	54	2	56	18	26	59	1	60	14	26
toilet not working or functioning badly	80	-	80	8	12	84	-	84	10	6
heating system not working or functioning badly	83	-	83	8	9	89	-	89	6	5
electrical system not working or working badly	87	-	87	6	7	95	-	95	3	2
Three Observations[a]										
window screens missing	91	-	91	5	4	88	1	89	8	3
window screens broken	60	6	66	23	22	69	7	76	17	7
wall and floor problems inside the house[b]	58	9	67	22	11	63	9	72	20	8
chipped paint outside house	57	11	68	22	10	56	8	64	25	11
gutters in poor condition	41	32	73	17	10	45	33	78	16	6

a. All information supplied by respondent; not interviewer observation.

b. Includes four separate problems: open cracks or holes in walls or ceilings, holes in the floor larger than size of a soda can top, broken plaster or chipped paint larger than about one square foot. Variable has value of one if any other of these problems is present.

85

closely resemble those of their nonelderly counterparts. The homes of both groups exhibited an impressive amount of structural problems at the start of the period. However, if the evidence on the persistency of various housing problems for which we have time series data is a guide, then it seems likely that these problems have been corrected once they were identified by their occupants. This pattern would be consistent with the high rate of repairs to the exterior of the dwellings observed earlier for the elderly.

It was suggested earlier that a dwelling's layout could strongly affect the need for households with an impaired member to make modifications to the unit. The lower panel of Table 4.5 gives some indicators of unit layout for the houses included in our sample. A surprisingly large share — almost 70% — have all of the living space on a single floor. Such a layout would certainly obviate the need for large modifications to place both a bedroom and bathroom on the lower floor in households where the stairs are a real impediment for one of its members. In addition, among multifloor units about 30% have both a bedroom and bath on the first floor. In short, the units in this sample have a remarkably good layout for accommodating persons with serious mobility limitations; and this may indeed help account for the low incidence of room changes toward bedrooms that was noted in the last section.[8]

LIVING ARRANGEMENT AND SOCIAL SUPPORT

This section covers several distinct areas related to living arrangements and the amount of support provided by family members. We begin with a description of the composition of the households included in our sample. This includes information on the principal activity of the head of household and spouse, if any, to give some idea of the amount of potential assistance available from these sources. We then turn to the frequency of contact between the head and spouse and children living outside of the home and number of organized social activities in which the head and spouse participate.

Living Arrangements

Basic demographic and employment information on the sample households, divided between those headed by a nonelderly person and those headed by an elderly person, is presented in Table 4.7. A glance at the table reveals several differences between the elderly households and their more youthful counterparts. Two differences are in the incidence of households being headed by a woman and in the structure of the households. At the end of the study period, a quarter of the nonelderly households were headed by women; fully 44% of elderly households were. These figures align nicely with only 6% of nonelderly households being women living alone, while 29% of elderly households were of this type. All together 35% of the elderly households in the sample are persons living alone—implying no potential assistance within the home.

There are two other large differences in household composition between the two groups. Among the elderly, families consisting of only a husband and wife are more common (29 vs. 13% at the end of the period); but husband-wife households with another adult (including children age 15 and over) are much more common among the nonelderly: 43 vs. 14% at the end of the period. This latter figure is itself sensitive to the age structure of the nonelderly sample. As noted in the last chapter, almost half of this group is headed by a person between 50 and 60 years of age; hence, many of these households have older teenage and college age children present.

There is a great deal of change in household composition ongoing over the study period. The most pervasive shifts are those associated with aging. The incidence of female household heads rises from 32 to 44% among older households. While the percentage of households constituted by single persons among the elderly rises from 25 to 35%, the share in two-person husband-wife households falls from 38 to 29%.

The figures in Tables 4.8 and 4.9 provide additional information on the extent of change going on within households over the five year period. The first row in Table 4.8 shows that a shift to female-headed status was nearly always permanent (i.e., most are in the one-time change category). In contrast, multiple changes in the number of people in the household were common; only 29% of the

TABLE 4.7

DEMOGRAPHIC ATTRIBUTES OF SAMPLE HOUSEHOLDS: WAVES 1-5
(percent)

Attribute	Non-elderly Headed Households					Elderly Headed Households				
	1	2	3	4	5	1	2	3	4	5
Female headed	20	22	24	24	25	32	36	39	43	44
3-5 persons	50	53	52	53	53	24	20	18	23	22
More than 5 persons	26	21	21	21	18	5	6	5	5	5
Activity of head										
- working	84	87	81	83	78	23	19	14	14	10
- retired, disabled	9	9	9	10	14	60	57	62	66	66
- keeping house	6	5	8	6	6	15	23	22	20	23
- going to school	-	-	-	-	-	-	1	-	-	1
Activity of spouse										
- working	51	44	44	48	46	22	22	13	13	13
- retired, disabled	1	3	1	4	4	20	26	28	23	31
- keeping house	46	51	52	48	47	54	48	53	60	53
- going to school	-	-	1	-	1	-	2	-	-	-
Boarder present	3	1	1	-	1	3	2	6	4	2

Household type										
- male living alone	2	4	4	3	4	5	7	7	7	6
- female living alone	4	5	6	7	6	20	21	25	27	29
- husband-wife only	9	10	8	8	13	38	35	33	27	29
- husband-wife w/other adult	43	44	46	48	43	17	16	15	17	14
- other	42	37	35	34	34	19	20	19	22	22

Changes Between Survey Waves

In head of house		6	4	2	2		4	5	4	1
In activity of head										
- more active		5	1	4	1		3	3	3	7
- less active		3	5	3	6		7	8	4	1
In activity of spouse										
- more active		3	7	6	4		3	1	2	1
- less active		7	6	4	5		3	6	2	2
In support in household composition										
- alone to multi-person		1	2	1	2		2	4	4	2
- husband-wife to h-w with adults		1	2	1	1		3	1	3	1
- "other" to husband-wife		6	6	4	2		1	2	1	1
Any change in household composition		17	19	10	12		18	20	18	14

TABLE 4.8

CHANGES IN HOUSEHOLD COMPOSITION, WAVES 1-5
(percents)

	Non-elderly Headed Households			Elderly Headed Households		
	No change	One-time change	Dynamic	No change	One-time change	Dynamic
Female head of household (5 obs.)	87	12	1	88	11	1
Changes between surveys (4 obs.):						
number of persons in household	29	25	46	48	24	28
household composition affecting extent of support	73	25	2	79	18	4
head of household	88	10	2	83	10	1

TABLE 4.9

SHIFT AMONG HOUSEHOLD TYPES OF ELDERLY HEADED
HOUSEHOLDS BETWEEN SURVEY WAVES 3 AND 4
(number of households)

Wave 3	Wave 4					
	male alone	female alone	H-w only	H-w and other adults	other	total
Male alone	11	0	0	0	2	13
Female alone	0	40	0	0	5	45
Husband-wife only	0	5	45	6	3	59
H-w plus other adults	0	0	3	22	.2	27
Other	1	3	0	2	27	33
Total	12	48	48	30	39	177

nonelderly households and 48% of the elderly had no change. Nearly half of the nonelderly and over a quarter of the elderly experienced more than one change in the number of persons in the home over the period. Many of these changes did not, however, effect the amount of support potentially available in the home, as indicated by the third row of figures in the table: only about a quarter of both elderly and nonelderly households experienced changes on this score.

A matrix of initial and final household types for the elderly households is provided in Table 4.9, using data from survey waves 3 and 4. These data, which are consistent with those for other periods, give an idea of the degree of change occurring. While most households experienced no change, some recorded substantial change. For example, seven persons went from living alone to being members of multiperson households, and nine persons made the change in the opposite direction. Five women were widowed or divorced. Six couples who had been living alone added another adult. In this single year 18% of these households changed their composition — an impressive amount of change, suggesting that the shifting of living arrangement to more supportive ones may be more feasible for many households than might otherwise be thought.

Substantial change was also occurring in the way in which many of these people spent their time. The second and third panels of data in Table 4.7 give percentage distributions of the principal activities of the head of house and the spouse, if any. By the end of the study period, when the youngest head of house among the elderly group was age 62, only 10% of the household heads were still reporting "working" as their primary activity, while 13% of the spouses did. Interestingly, working also declined among the nonelderly: heads reported to be working falling from 84 to 78% and spouses from 51 to 46%. Again, this is presumably influenced by the age structure of our nonelderly sample.

Two lower panels in the table classify the year-to-year changes in the activity of heads and spouses into "more active" and "less active" groups. Shifting from retirement to work or school are both classified as "more active," for example. Among the nonelderly the pattern is rather mixed with fairly balanced changes in both directions. Among the elderly, however, the pattern is more dominantly one of reduced activity levels.

The overall picture of the older households included in this study that emerges from these data is definitely one of aging, as indicated by reduced working, the rise in single person households, and the decline in the incidence of simple husband-wife households. On the other hand, all of the information points to many households experiencing a great deal of churning in living arrangements and the number of persons present in the household from year-to-year. The dynamism of these arrangements suggest considerable potential opportunity for changing to more supportive environments by those who need to do so.

Other Social Contacts

While living arrangements are extremely important in determining the amount of social support and assistance with everyday activities a person might receive, there are certainly other ways of obtaining some of these "services." The survey administered to the sample households inquired extensively about the contact of the respondent and spouse with children who were no longer living at home and about their organized social activities. The questionnaire did not cover informal social contacts. (Later in this chapter we will discuss the amount of assistance with activities of daily living these households received and who provided it.)

The data in Table 4.10 inform us that three out of every four elderly households had at least one child living outside their homes; the rate for the nonelderly was about two out of three by the end of the period. Both groups of parents had a great deal of contact with their children: two-thirds see a child at least weekly and three-fourths talk to a child weekly. Only about 9% of the elderly do not talk to a child at least monthly and around 20% do not see a child at least monthly.

Presumably these frequent contacts, especially the visits, are dependent on the proximity of the children. The figures in the table confirm the almost amazing proximity of at least one child to his parents: about one-third of the parents have a child living in their own neighborhood and about 70% have a child within an hour's car drive of their home.[9]

Interestingly, an examination of cross-tabulations of the frequency of contact and the proximity of children to their parents does not provide support for the hypothesis that elderly living alone have more contact and live closer to their children than elderly living in multiperson households.

The data presented in Table 4.11 show that the frequency of contact was very stable over the observation period, especially among the elderly. The great majority of those reporting frequent contact in one survey also did so in the other two surveys in which these questions were asked. It is important to note that these frequent contacts with children persisted despite a good deal of residential mobility on the part of the children, as shown in the fifth and sixth rows of figures in the table. Among the elderly only 19% had children living in their neighborhood for the entire period, although nearly one-third reported having a child in the neighborhood in each survey wave. As one would expect, there is greater stability among children being within an hour of their parent's home.

In terms of organized activities outside of the home, church attendance is by far the most important. Sixty percent of the elderly declared themselves as "regular" attendees in each survey wave. In contrast, 16% or less reported themselves as involved in another type of regular activity, including participation in a neighborhood

TABLE 4.10

INCIDENCE OF SOCIAL ACTIVITIES AND SUPPORT
(percent)

	Non-Elderly Headed			Elderly Headed		
	W3	W4	W5	W3	W4	W5
Relations with Children:						
No children outside of home	41	35	34	24	24	24
For those w/kids living away:						
see one at least weekly	67	73	72	66	66	71
do not see even monthly	15	17	13	23	20	13
talk to one at least weekly	76	77	72	75	74	79
do not talk to them even monthly	6	11	15	9	9	10
at least one lives in neighborhood	31	27	24	33	26	33
at least one lives within hour's drive[a]	67	75	74	71	77	76
Participation in local activities:[b]						
Some activity regularly	19	15	15	16	10	14
Two or more activities "sometimes"[c]	3	3	4	-	1	1
Any activity "sometimes"[c]	16	13	13	8	9	7
Church attendance:						
Regularly attends	55	54	53	60	59	58
Sometimes attends	38	39	39	29	29	28

a. Not the same child as the one living in the neighborhood, if any.
b. Respondent was prompted on neighborhood associations, political clubs, recreation groups (such as bridge, quilting, softball, bowling).
c. Does no activity regularly.

TABLE 4.11

CONSISTENCY OF CONTACTS WITH CHILDREN, WAVES 3-5[a]
(percents)

| | Non-elderly Headed Households | | | | | Elderly Headed Households | | | | |
| | stable | | | one-time | | stable | | | one-time | |
	high	low	total	shift	dynamic	high	low	total	shift	dynamic
Contact with children:										
see one at least weekly	58	16	74	15	11	58	19b	77	10	13
do not see one even monthly	76	8b	84	10	6	74	10b	84	10	6
talk to one at least weekly	55	6	61	15	24	62	10	72	13	15
do not talk to one even monthly	82	2	84	11	5	84	2	86	8	6
at least one lives in the neighborhood	10	52	62	25	13	19	55	74	14	12
at least one lives within an hour's drive	54	10	64	12	24	62	10	72	13	15
Participation in local activities:										
some activity regularly	5	68	73	20	7	4	75	79	14	7
two or more activities "sometimes"	1	91	92	7	1	-	98	98	2	-
attend church regularly	45	22	77	7	16	45	28	73	16	11

a. Samples restricted to households with at least one child living outside of the home throughout the period.
b. To clarify the definition: this entry means the parent does not see child monthly.

95

association, political club, or various recreation groups (bowling, quilting, etc.). When one examines the persistence of participation in these activities (Table 4.11), one sees that except for attending church almost no one participates year after year in another activity. While there is some flux even among church-goers, nearly half of all the elderly responded that they attended church in all three survey waves.

We hypothesized for the elderly living alone, that those without children would be more active in neighborhood and church functions—the idea being that those without children would use such activities to compensate for the absence of interactions with children. However, an examination of the relevant cross-tabulations provided no support for this hypothesis.

The elderly have a wide-range of contacts which stimulate them and which can be a source of help when needed, either on an episodic or continuous basis. Among these contacts, those through church and those with their children are clearly paramount, if regularity and frequency of interaction is a reliable measure in this regard. Of course, the arrangements in which they live probably dominate any interactions outside of the home. The large number of elderly living alone are clearly at a disadvantage; doubly disadvantaged are those who live alone and who do not have children. These are important exceptions to the more frequent situation characterized by a variety of contacts within and outside the home.

ACTIVITY LIMITATIONS

Differences between the nonelderly and the elderly in the extent of activity limitations and the corresponding amount of help the two groups receive with activities of daily living are well-documented. We expect these differences to be important in distinguishing the types of housing adjustments made by nonelderly and elderly headed households. This section provides an introduction to the problems the households in our sample have with performing certain actions and the amount of help they obtain with daily tasks.

Activity Limitations

For the third through fifth waves of the household survey of the sample, a separate battery of questions was included on the activity limitations of the respondent and the spouse or partner (if any). Inquiries were made about 11 specific types of limitations; for each one that the respondent indicated was a problem, the survey asked when it first became a problem and then asked whether the person has the problem "all the time, some of the time, or occasionally?"[10] Information on the use of canes, walkers, and wheelchairs was also obtained. For our analysis we have compressed the 11 categories into the six shown in the left-hand stub of Table 4.12.

The figures in the table show several interesting patterns. First, the major difference in the incidence of activity limitations is, as expected, between the nonelderly and the elderly. Respondents and spouses in the two groups report remarkably similar levels of limitations. This is perhaps most easily seen in the "weighted sum of activity limitations" figures. This measure, defined in the notes to the table, weights each problem reported by the frequency of its occurrence. Among the nonelderly both respondents and spouses have scores in the 15-20 range, while the elderly have scores at least three times as great in the 60-70 range.

The most frequently reported limitations are (a) gardening or using a step stool and (b) restricted mobility in or outside of the home. At least 30% of the elderly report such problems. After these, problems with hearing and seeing are the greatest.[11] The elderly report a substantial incidence in the use of aids in getting about. Depending on the data for which year is used, on the order of 15% of respondents and 9% of spouses use such devices overall, and perhaps one-third of these are using wheelchairs.

The data in Table 4.12 show a fair amount of year-to-year change in the incidence of individual limitations. Since in doing the surveys it was possible for the respondent not to be the same person in each wave (although it had to be the head or spouse), some of the variation may come from this source. In examining the persistence of reported problems over the three waves we have, therefore, restricted the sample to those cases in which the respondent was the same person in all three waves in which there was no change on the

TABLE 4.12

INCIDENCE OF ACTIVITY LIMITATIONS: WAVES 3-5
(percents)

	Non-elderly Headed Households			Elderly Headed Households		
	W3	W4	W5	W3	W4	W5
Respondent						
Has following activity limitations:						
1. mobility in or outside of home	1	5	4	16	15	14
2. using bathroom, grasping faucets	3	5	4	4	7	8
3. getting in/out of bed, dressing	2	3	2	5	7	6
4. doing gardening, using step stool	14	9	7	29	30	27
5. hearing	4	3	1	17	12	8
6. seeing	2	4	3	10	9	7
Weighted sum of limitations[a]	20	19	15	70	69	61
Use special equipment to get around	3	3	4	16	12	18
of this group, % using wheelchair	-	-	-	40	50	25
Spouse[b]						
Has following activity limitations:						
1. mobility in or outside of home	2	3	3	16	17	15
2. using bathroom, grasping faucets	2	2	3	7	10	9
3. getting in/out of bed, dressing	2	3	2	6	6	10
4. doing gardening, using step stool	8	9	6	21	22	23
5. hearing	2	2	2	10	10	4
6. seeing	5	5	1	8	10	5
Weighted sum of limitations[a]	18	17	14	60	68	62
Use special equipment to get around	2	6	3	9	9	9
of this group, % using wheelchair	-	-	100	-	67	50
Spouse present	68	68	68	50	46	44

a. Weights are frequency of occurrence: 3 = all of the time; 2 = most of the time; 1 = occasionally.
Index = [(problem reported * weight)/(no. of problems reported * 3)] * 100, where problem reported equals 1 if a problem is reported and 0 if a problem is not reported.
b. All calculations based on spouses only.

head or spouse over the observation period. (Some 35 of the 177 households in the elderly sample are lost when this is done.) Table 4.13 shows the percentage of these individuals in our sample of households headed by an elderly person reporting a particular problem in all three survey waves, in no waves, or in one or two waves. (This last group is labeled "other" in the table.) The table includes separate tabulations for those respondents living alone and those in multiperson households.

The startling pattern in these figures is the small percentage of persons persistently reporting a problem. Depending on the particular measure examined, only about one-fourth to one-half of the persons reporting a problem in any year are seen to report it over a three year period. For example, among respondents, 13% report having trouble doing gardening or using a step stool in all three waves; but in the individual surveys 27 to 30% report this as a problem. It is likely that the low share of those persistently reporting a limitation is in part due to some limitations only beginning after the start of the period. Even so, these percentages seem surprisingly low.

It is possible to obtain some idea of how large a "pool" of respondents those reporting a problem on a yearly basis are drawn by adding those reporting it as a problem every year to those reporting it as a problem in one or two years. To continue the example with those having problems with gardening and using a step stool, one sees that 50% report this as a problem at any time (13 plus 37, in the first set of columns in Table 4.13). Thus the pool of those "ever reporting" the problem is not quite double those reporting it as a problem yearly and about three times those reporting it all three years. There is some variance in these ratios among the individual activity limitations — especially for limitations regarding use of the bathroom and getting in and out of bed. Still, these parameters are in fact reasonably serviceable for respondents as orders of magnitude for the relationship among problems reported yearly, those which are persistently reported, and all of those ever reporting a specific problem. To present these figures somewhat differently, if one knows the percentage of persons reporting a problem in a given

TABLE 4.13

STABILITY OF REPORTED ACTIVITY LIMITATIONS AMONG THE ELDERLY, WAVES 3-5, BY HOUSEHOLD TYPE

(percents)

Respondent Has following activity limitations:	All elderly stable high	All elderly stable low	All elderly total	All elderly other	Elderly living alone stable high	Elderly living alone stable low	Elderly living alone total	Elderly living alone other	Elderly living with others stable high	Elderly living with others stable low	Elderly living with others total	Elderly living with others other
1. mobility inside or outside of home	6	72	78	22	8	69	77	23	4	74	78	22
2. using bathroom	1	85	86	14	2	84	86	14	0	86	86	14
3. getting in/out of bed, dressing	1	87	88	12	2	88	90	10	1	86	87	13
4. doing gardening, using step stool	13	50	63	37	12	51	63	27	13	49	62	38
5. hearing	6	77	83	17	8	67	75	25	4	82	86	14
6. seeing	4	81	85	15	4	78	82	19	3	48	51	49
Using special equipment to get around												
- any	10	75	85	15	14	71	85	15	8	76	84	16
- wheelchair[e]	1	98	99	1	0	100	100	-	1	63	64	36
(n)	(142)				(49)				(93)			

Spouse[c] Has following activity limitations:				[d]
1. mobility inside or outside of home	3	45	48	52
2. using bathroom	3	57	60	40
3. getting in/out of bed, dressing	3	57	60	40
4. doing gardening, using step stool	6	43	49	51
5. hearing	3	59	60	40
6. seeing	5	60	65	35
Using special equipment to get around				
- any	3	56	59	41
- wheelchair[e]	-	65	65	35
(n)	(56)			

a. Population restricted to households with no change in head or spouse over period and in which respondent was always the same person.
b. Has problem every period.
c. Population is spouses present.
d. Same as entries in first 4 columns.
e. Of those using any special equipment.

year, then it is likely that he is drawn from a "pool" of persons about twice as great who would report the problem in some year and only about one-third of those reporting it in this year will report the problem every year for three years.

These ratios do *not* hold for spouses, who are women only about 40% of the time, i.e., the woman was normally the respondent in a husband-wife household.[12] (The structure of the survey and coding of the data make it inadvisable to disregard the identity of the respondent as such and label each person as husband or wife.) The percentage of spouses indicating persistent problems is lower than for the respondents, and those reporting a problem in any year are drawn from much larger "pools" than are the respondents. Indeed the pools for spouses included from 40 to 55% of all spouses, compared with 13 to 50% for respondents. In short, spouses appear to have these problems on a significantly more episodic basis than respondents.[13]

Another interesting pattern revealed by the data in Table 4.13 is the little difference between the incidence of persistence between those elderly living alone and those in multiperson households. Indeed, there are only two limitations for which those living alone report lower persistence than those living in other arrangements. This similarity of the two groups is contrary to our expectations. Based on analyses of the determinants of institutionalization, we expected lower rates for those living alone. It may be that these persons are receiving sufficient assistance from outside of the home or have made changes to their dwelling to offset the comparative difficulties of living alone.

We can obtain some idea of the relationship between making modifications to the dwelling to compensate for activity limitations and the presence of such limitations through a simple cross-tabulation. The tabulation is of the activity limitation score measure (discussed above) computed for the respondent and the presence of modifications. The score measure is used as it captures intensity as well as presence of problems. The figures reported in Table 4.14 are for all respondents in elderly headed households as of the third household survey wave. (Small counts of modifications prevented us from doing similar computations only for those living alone.) Tabulations for all modifications and for moderate modifications

TABLE 4.14

Relationship Between Activity Limitations of Respondent and
the Presence of Dwelling Modifications for
Elderly-Headed Households at Wave 3

Activity Limitation Score[a]	% of Households Reporting Any Modification[b]	Moderate Modifications
Under 50	13	12
50-100	17	17
100-150	13	-
150-200	31	31
over 200	55	38

a. For respondent; see note to Table 4.12 for definition.
b. See notes to Table 4.1 for definitions.

(the most populous subcategory) are shown. The data exhibit a fairly clear pattern in which the presence of at least one modification is found more often as the activity limitations of the respondent increase in number and intensity. Thus, while the installation of such modifications may be comprised of highly discrete events, there is clear evidence that the presence of modifications is related to activity limitations.[14]

Supportive Services

Beginning with the third household survey, the interview instrument included a battery of questions on whether the respondent or spouse received help with 10 different activities of daily living. It did not ask if the person needed help with each activity. If receipt of help was reported, follow up questions asked who provided it (someone inside the home, if outside the home the relationship of the person to the household or whether an agency was the provider), when help was first received, whether it was usually paid for, and whether they were still receiving it. While the responses to these questions have provided a great deal of useful information, we have discovered in the analysis that some problems are apparently present. In particular, in the responses about the spouse, the respondents often answered that the spouse received help. Given the frequency of these responses and the fact that almost all of the help came from within the household, our image is of most responses indicating someone else in the household "helping out" in contrast to providing compensating assistance.

Basic figures on the receipt of supportive services are given in Table 4.15, for nonelderly and elderly households. These figures are for wave 3; data from other waves are similar. The 10 individual types of assistance which were inquired about are listed in the left-hand stub along with some summary measures. For the reasons outlined above, we concentrate on the responses for the respondents. The overall incidence of help received is about the same for nonelderly and elderly. However, the elderly report sharply higher rates of obtaining assistance from sources outside of the home and of paying for it. (The figures on help outside the home and paid help are computed as percentages of those receiving some help.) For example, for heavy housework, 25% of the nonelderly and 32% of the elderly report receiving some help; for the nonelderly only 9% of those receiving help obtain it from outside the home, while 52% of the elderly obtain it from external sources. None of the nonelderly pay for such help but 11% of the elderly receiving such help do so.

Even with their greater assistance from outside of the home, the elderly still obtain a great deal of help from within the household — from one-half to two-thirds of assistance comes from within the home. The highest rates of assistance from outside the home are for managing money and grocery shopping; the next group is heavy housework, personal needs (bathing, etc.), and help when sick; the third high incidence group is for light housework and laundry. Aside from personal needs for which very few respondents report receiving help, the highest incidence of payment for services is for doing light housework and laundry, i.e., maid services.

The average respondent in an elderly headed household received assistance with 1.55 of the 10 tasks. Of these about half were obtained from outside the home. Of all the tasks for which help was received, only about 10% were paid for.

Data on the persistence with which assistance was received are presented in Table 4.16. We saw earlier that the persistence of activity limitations is quite small compared to the annual rates; and we should expect, therefore, that receipt of assistance would exhibit a similar pattern. Again concentrating on the figures for households headed by an elderly person in the lower panel of the table, we see that this expectation is supported. Generally the percentage of respondents reporting receiving assistance during all three periods is about half that reporting receiving assistance in a single year. Likewise, the total volume of households receiving assistance any time over the period (the sum of those receiving it every year and those receiving it one or two years) is typically about 50% larger than those obtaining assistance in a single year.

Sharply different patterns from these are displayed for obtaining help from outside the home and paying for help. For these groups the ratio of the percentage of households persistently receiving help to the percentage receiving help in a single year is much lower than the similar ratio for obtaining help from any source. To take preparing meals as an example, for assistance from any source the ratio of those receiving help in all three years to those receiving it one or two years is 8:22; for those receiving it from outside the home, the ratio is 1:12. The percentage of households reporting receiving assistance persistently is only one-fourth to one-sixth as large as those receiving such assistance in a given year. This pattern holds across all of the types of assistance covered. The unmistakable conclusion is that help outside of the home is only turned to as a necessity and it is very hard to sustain such assistance — either because volunteers cannot sustain their efforts or because households cannot afford the expense of paid assistance.

We have explored somewhat further the relationship between the persistency of receiving help from any source and the persistency of paying for help. Data on this point are presented in Table 4.17. The figures in the table are *counts* of respondents in each category. Thus, for example, 11 respondents reported receiving help in all three waves in preparing meals. Of these, nine never paid for help and two paid for help in one or two of the observation periods. Across the 10 types of tasks inquired about, there were only four households who reported paying for help in all three waves and these paid for housework and laundry services. An examination of the figures in the last column reinforces the pattern of infrequency with which such services are purchased. In sum, payment for these

TABLE 4.15

Help Received with Activities of Daily Living at Wave 3

	Non-Elderly Headed Households			Elderly Headed Households		
	Receives some help	help from outside home[b]	paid help[b]	receives some help	help from outside home[b]	paid help[b]
Respondent						
Individual help items:						
preparing meals	15%	14%	7%	15%	19%	7%
laundry	20	3	5	20	39	19
light housework	22	19	4	21	37	16
heavy housework	25	9	-	32	52	11
making phone calls	2	33	2	4	29	-
grocery shopping	26	8	-	33	58	7
help when sick	16	27	-	18	48	3
managing money	14	4	-	10	59	-
personal needs	3	40	-	1	50	50
moving inside house	2	50	-	1	50	-
Summary measures[a]						
No. of services received	1.45			1.55		
No. of services provided by persons from outside the home	.19			.70		
No. of services paid for	.03			.15		

Spouse
Individual help items:

preparing meals	39	2	–	31	–	–
laundry	39	2	–	31	4	4
light housework	40	2	–	34	3	3
heavy housework	38	2	–	42	11	3
making phone calls	6	2	–	12	–	–
grocery shopping	36	–	–	40	11	–
help when sick	24	–	–	26	9	–
managing money	31	3	–	30	11	0
personal needs	1	–	–	6	–	–
moving inside house	2	–	–	4	–	–
Summary measures[a]						
No. of services received	1.79			1.29		
No. of services provided by persons from outside the home	.02			.08		
No. of services paid for	-			.02		

a. Defined for all households. So, number of services received, for example, is for all households not just those saying they need some service.
b. Computed as percentage of those receiving help.

107

TABLE 4.16

Persistence of the Receipt of Help by Respondents, Waves 3-5[a]
(percents)

Group and Type of Help Received	Receives some help stable high[c]	low[d]	total	other[e]	Help from outside home stable high	low	total	other	Help is paid for stable high	low	total	other
Non-elderly Headed Households												
preparing meals	6	69	75	25	–	97	97	3	–	98	98	2
laundry	7	66	73	27	–	97	97	3	–	97	97	3
light housework	11	60	71	29	–	94	94	6	–	97	97	3
heavy housework	11	55	66	34	–	92	92	8	–	95	95	5
making phone calls	–	91	91	9	–	99	99	1	–	100	100	1
grocery shopping	9	62	71	29	–	97	97	3	–	99	99	1
help when sick	3	77	78	22	1	95	96	4	–	99	99	1
managing money	3	74	77	23	–	100	100	–	–	100	100	–
personal needs	–	96	96	4	–	99	99	1	–	100	100	–
moving inside house	–	95	95	5	–	99	99	1	–	100	100	–
Elderly Headed Households												
preparing meals	8	70	78	22	1	87	88	12	2	97	99	1
laundry	13	66	79	21	5	83	88	12	1	92	93	7
light housework	10	65	75	25	2	84	86	14	1	94	95	5
heavy housework	17	51	68	32	8	73	81	19	1	92	93	7
making phone calls	1	94	95	5	–	97	97	3	1	99	99	1
grocery shopping	20	50	70	30	8	65	73	27	1	95	96	4
help when sick	6	71	77	23	3	81	84	16	–	97	97	3
managing money	6	80	86	14	2	89	91	9	–	99	99	1
personal needs	1	94	95	5	1	96	97	3	–	99	99	1
moving inside house	1	96	97	3	–	98	98	2	–	100	100	–

a. See Table 4.13 for definition of respondents included in this analysis. All computations are for the full population.

b. Persons living outside of the respondent's home; includes public agencies and paid-for help.

c. Received help every year.

d. Never received help.

e. Received help in one or two years.

TABLE 4.17

Number of Elderly Respondents Who Reported Receiving Help in
All Waves (3-5) by Persistence of Paying for Such Help
(counts)

Assisted Task	Total	high[a]	Stable low[b]	total	other[c]
preparing meals	11	-	9	9	2
laundry	18	2	13	15	3
light housework	14	-	10	10	4
heavy housework	24	2	16	18	6
making phone calls	1	-	1	1	-
grocery shopping	29	-	26	26	3
help when sick	9	-	8	8	1
managing money	8	-	8	8	-
personal needs	1	-	-	-	1
moving inside house	1	-	1	1	-

a. Paid for help in every period.
b. Never paid for help.
c. Paid for help in one or two periods.

types of services is in general a rare event and persistent payment for them, even among those receiving services consistently, almost nonexistent.

A remaining question concerns the relationship between the presence of activity limitations and the receipt of supportive services of various types. Although the surveys did not make a close linkage between these two domains in the actual sequence of questions, there are clear logical connections between certain limitations and types of assistance that could be required. Mobility limitations, for instance, could necessitate help with a number of the tasks about which we inquired—such as housework, grocery shopping, and moving inside the dwelling. Table 4.18 presents cross-tabulations of the activity limitations by type of assistance received for the respondents in elderly headed households; separate figures are provided for persons living alone and those in multiperson households. The population is different for each column in the table, i.e., for each activity limitation the population is comprised of those reporting this activity limitation at the time of the third household survey. The number of persons in these populations is small (see the final

TABLE 4.18

Percentage of Elderly Household Respondents with Each Activity Limitation Who Receive Some Help by Living Arrangement[a,e]

	Activity limitation							
	lives alone				lives with others			
Type of help received	mobility	gardening[f]	hearing	seeing	mobility	gardening[f]	hearing	seeing
preparing meals	20[b]	13	—	d	16(11)[c]	17(10)	61(6)	42(16)
laundry	40	30	23		27(16)	23(10)	41(12)	50(16)
light housework	50	39	23		38(16)	27(10)	41(18)	33(16)
heavy housework	60	56	31		49(22)	61(24)	52(29)	50(16)
making phone calls	—	—	8		11(5)	13(3)	12(6)	25(8)
grocery shopping	100	61	38		61(33)	51(21)	28(12)	50(25)
help when sick	30	22	23		33(28)	31(24)	29(12)	50(25)
managing money	30	13	—		27(22)	27(17)	17(12)	25(16)
personal needs	10	4	—		5(0)	—	—	8(0)
moving inside house	—	—	—		5(0)	3(—)	—	8(0)
n	10	23	13		18	29	17	12

a. Data from household survey wave 3.

b. Population in this cell is the elderly respondents who reported a mobility limitation in wave 3 who lived alone. Twenty percent of this group received help preparing meals.

c. Figure in parentheses is the percent of households who received help from outside the home. By definition all help provided to those living alone came from outside of the home.

d. Not tabulated; number reporting problem is less than 10.

e. Limitations in use of bathrooms, etc. and getting in and out of bed are not included because the sample sizes are too small.

f. Includes use of step stool as well as gardening.

row of the table); and the patterns shown should be taken as no more than suggestive.

The overall pattern is that the majority of households needing assistance seem to be receiving it. The difference between the two groups of households are not pronounced, with the possible exception for those reporting mobility limitations, for whom those living alone receive a somewhat higher volume of assistance in general. For those with this limitation help with grocery shopping and housework seem to be especially important. The pattern of assistance received for those having problems with gardening or using a step stool are similar to those with other mobility limitations, as one would expect. Those with hearing and seeing problems both obtain help with a wide range of tasks.

Lastly note that for multiperson households the figures in parentheses indicate the percentage of assistance received from outside of the home. Two points are of interest. First, almost universally a substantial portion of all assistance received is from outside the home. Thus, the importance of external support is by no means limited to those living alone. Second, as one would expect, the share of services provided from outside the home is consistently lower for those in multiperson households than for those living alone.

A final area of supportive services to be covered is the participation of the sample households in certain formal support programs. In particular, we inquired about receipt of meals, attendance at senior centers, and the use of transportation services. Use of such services reduces the need for other kinds of support and therefore information about them is needed to help provide a complete picture of the resources used by the sample households. Table 4.19 summarizes the utilization of these three types of services. Overall, around 20% of the sample households use one of these services. A nontrivial percentage of elderly headed households receive meals in their homes or attend senior citizen centers on a regular basis—about 7% in each group. A similar number makes use of transportation services. These figures suggest that such services are an important complement to other supportive services received. On the other hand, almost none of these households use these services year after year.

TABLE 4.19

Receipt of Other Support Services: Waves 3-5
(percent)

	Non-elderly Headed Household			Elderly Headed Household		
	W3	W4	W5	W3	W4	W5
Meals received						
regularly	-	-	-	4	6	7
occasionally	2	1	1	2	1	1
Attends center for adults						
regularly	2	1	1	7	7	10
occasionally	1	2	3	2	6	3
Transportation services received?	2	1	1	8	7	6

The data reviewed on activity limitations and supportive services paint a remarkably consistent picture for households headed by an elderly person. In any year a substantial share of respondents and spouses report activity limitations; and each year most receive some assistance in coping with these limitations, very often from sources outside of the home. At the same time the persistence of these activity limitations — in the sense of their being reported successively over a three year period — is quite low. Only for gardening and using a step stool do as many as 10% of respondents report a persistent problem. Likewise, the persistent receipt of assistance with various tasks of daily living from outside of the home (especially services paid for) is extremely rare. The pattern is definitely one of episodic problems and corresponding responses. Apparently those with more serious and persistent problems are unable to remain in their homes and either move to more supportive environments in the community or shift to institutions.

ECONOMIC POSITION

Since the economic position of American households is quite well-documented, we reviewed briefly and selectively the general information on this topic gathered in our surveys.[15] Our focus is on the dynamics of income and wealth, in part because the studies reviewed in Chapter 2 point to considerable income change surrounding the act of retirement.

Summary data for the five survey waves are provided separately for households headed by a nonelderly person and those with elderly heads in Table 4.20. In comparing the figures for the two groups of households it is important to recall that both groups are drawn from the same neighborhoods. Hence, given the homogeneity of neighborhoods in American cities, one expects the general economic attributes of the elderly and nonelderly to be similar. With respect to total household income, the anticipated higher level for the nonelderly compared to the elderly is present. But the growth in incomes of the two groups over the five year period has been quite similar: 34% for the nonelderly households and 28% for the elderly.

The value of home equity reported by the two groups is also quite

TABLE 4.20

Income, Assets, and Housing Expenses: Waves 1-5

	Non-elderly Headed Households					Elderly Headed Households				
	1	2	3	4	5	1	2	3	4	5
Annual total income ($000s)	13.9	16.3	17.8	17.9	18.6	8.0	7.8	9.3	9.7	10.2
Home equity ($000s)	18.9	23.1	25.4	26.5	26.7	23.2	26.9	29.4	28.7	26.8
Net wealth ($000s)	22.4	27.5	29.3	31.8	30.2	29.7	34.5	34.1	35.3	30.2
Mortgage, property tax, insurance monthly payments ($)	127	145	136	139	140	61	70	54	53	56
Fixed obligations[a] ($)	223	276	319	286	295	134	175	167	174	178
Disposable income/total income[b] (percent)	75	72	75	72	75	71	64	72	71	72
No debt on home (percent)	41	40	34	32	34	76	80	74	73	76

a. Fixed obligations include payments for mortgages, property taxes, homeowners insurance, utilities, alimony, and child support.
b. Disposable income is total income less fixed obligations.

114

similar, and in both cases home equity accounts for the great majority of net wealth holdings. The similarity in home equity holdings is somewhat surprising because a much higher share of the elderly do not have any debt on their homes (about 75 vs. 35%). The similarity may mean that the nonelderly systematically occupy better or larger homes, but there is nothing in our data that supports this idea; an alternative explanation is simply that the elderly are underestimating their equity position.

A final note of interest regarding home equity is the pattern of increases in the average values over time. The sharply rising property values at the end of the 1970s is evident in the values for the first three survey waves. For the latter part of the observation period, however, the pause in the growth of property values is clear. This pause was caused by the combination of the recession, extremely high real mortgage interest rates, and the reduction in marginal federal income tax rates enacted in 1981 which reduced the value of tax deductions associated with homeownership.

The figures on housing expenses, fixed obligations, and disposable income (the latter defined as the income available after paying for housing and other fixed expenses) are of interest primarily for what they tell us about the extent that families' other consumption is being constrained by such obligations. The figures in the table show that the average ratio of disposable to total income is the same for the two groups of households at about 72-75%. The similarity in ratios results from the housing expenses of the elderly being relatively low in absolute terms because so many own their homes free-and-clear of mortgage debt. This offsets the effect of their lower incomes; that is, both the numerator and the denominator in the ratio of disposable to total income is lower for the elderly than for the nonelderly. Thus, on an average basis the elderly have the same share of their income available for "discretionary" spending. Moreover, an examination of the distributions of this ratio for the two groups show the distributions to be quite similar. The principal difference is that fewer of the elderly are in the highest ratio categories: presumably the nonelderly in this group are those with no mortgage debt and high preretirement incomes.[16]

While not explored here in detail, it is worth noting that there is not a very close relationship between a household's income and its net wealth position among our sample households (see Annex table C.2). On the other hand, there is a close correspondence between gross and disposable incomes.

An issue of particular concern for this study is the extent of change in household incomes and wealth over time. An effective way to study such changes is to categorize financial variables into quartiles each year and to examine the extent to which households move between such quartiles over time. We expect that income changes among the elderly will be greater than those among the nonelderly because of the sharp reductions in incomes that accompany widowhood and retirement, the considerable number of retirements that occurred, and the number of women who were widowed among our sample households over the period.

We have done the type of analysis just outlined for total household income and net wealth, and the results are shown in Table 4.21. Most of the entries report changes between successive survey waves ("wave-to-wave" changes). Two numbers are reported for each pair of waves: the first is the percentage of all households that remained in the same quartile in both waves; the second is the percentage of households that moved more than one income quartile between the two waves, e.g., Q4 to Q1. The figures show remarkable stability, especially for total income, after allowing for noise from reporting errors and imputations." Consistently 60% of households, both nonelderly and elderly are in the same quartile in both periods. Only between the first two waves do as many as 10% of households shift by more than one quartile. Generally about a quarter of all households move a single income quartile between periods. We can only speculate on why the patterns are so similar for the two groups. One explanation is that loss of work during the recession was quite important for the nonelderly; but this seems unsatisfactory because the figures in Table 4.7 show the elderly leaving the labor force at a much higher rate than the nonelderly. Another explanation might involve reduced hours of work during the recession. But none of these explanations is very convincing.

The final row of the table reports the change over five survey waves in the income positions of respondents using the same measures. Forty-six percent of nonelderly and elderly households are in the same income quartile at the end of the period as they were at the

TABLE 4.21

Summary of Relative Changes in Financial Position Between Survey Waves

	Non-elderly Headed Households		Elderly-headed Households	
	in same quartile	more than 1 quartile change	in same quartile	more than 1 quartile change
Wave to Wave Changes				
Total income				
W1-2	60	10	67	10
2-3	53	7	50	8
3-4	60	4	63	7
4-5	52	6	61	4
Net wealth				
W1-2	60	4	57	10
2-3	48	9	50	9
3-4	57	6	59	5
4-5	66	6	64	8
First wave vs. last wave				
Total income	46	19	46	13

a. Elderly and non-elderly households classified separately into quartiles for each survey wave.

start. On the other hand, nearly one in five have shifted position by more than one quartile. These figures indicate substantial income mobility (both positive and negative) by a significant portion of the population over this five year period.

Overall these data point to considerable stability in the economic positions of households, while at the same time exhibiting a significant amount of shifting from year-to-year and rather more across several years. This degree of income variation could certainly affect the timing of undertaking major modifications or improvements to a family's home or cause it to consider taking in boarders to supplement income.

NOTES

1. This data set is rather susceptible to reporting errors because we did not require that the same persons act as the respondent for each survey; in about 80% of the cases the respondent was the same, at least for the last three household surveys. Reporting problems seem especially likely when the respondent answered questions about the spouse's activity limitations and need for help.

2. We have information for five survey waves on repairs and improvements and on the presence of boarders, but only for three waves on the other topics.

3. This pattern is not shown in Table 4.2; it was present in the detailed listing of the patterns of change over time described earlier (i.e., the XOX data).

4. For data for the elderly and nonelderly separately on this point, see Struyk and Soldo (1980), Tables 4.1 and 4.2. After adjusting the 1977 figures reported there for the elderly for inflation to 1982, they yield an annual average expenditure figure for all households of about $200. Nineteen eighty-two corresponds to the time covered by our fourth survey period.

5. There is only a weak relationship between the number of major modifications to the unit reported in any period and the number of major repairs or renovations reported, thus indicating that most of these major improvements are not associated with adjusting the home for use of an impaired person.

6. See Table C.1 for these results.

7. At the other end of the range, 3% of the units occupied by nonelderly and 6% of those occupied by the elderly were observed to have three or more structural problems.

8. We computed cross-tabulations of different types of room changes in multistory units against the types of rooms that were on the first floor. The number of observations was very small and no clear patterns were evident.

9. More specifically, of those seeing a child at least monthly, 37% have a child living in their neighborhood and 69% have at least one child living within an hour's car drive.

10. In wave 3, the first in which such questions were asked, the date when the problem first occurred was asked. In the subsequent waves, the questions were directed to problems that had arisen since the last survey. In practice there was a good deal of overlap in the problems reported in the various waves, and for practical purposes each wave can be thought of asking about problems present at that time.

11. The incidence rates shown for the elderly are somewhat higher than those reviewed in Chapter 2 based on a national sample. The interested reader should compare the figures in Table 2.4 with those in Tables 4.12 and 4.15.

12. While we have not been able to verify this with our data, it may be that in a number of cases the less frail person acted as the respondent in husband-wife households. This may account for some findings in the next chapter in which limitations on the part of the spouse are especially important.

13. We had hoped to examine those multiperson households in which both the respondent and spouse reported an activity limitation. The sample available, however, was simply too small: only 15 households reported the presence of an activity limitation by both persons.

14. This is consistent with the evidence cited in Chapter 2 from earlier studies.

15. We needed more of these data than we discussed at this point in order to construct a full description in this domain of the sample households for the multivariate analysis.

16. See Table C.4.

17. The largest numbers of values had to be imputed for the financial variables, especially incomes of all the domains. For a further explanation of imputation procedures see Appendix B.

Chapter 5

Multivariate Analysis

This chapter presents our analysis of causal relationships determining the type and extent of in-place housing adjustments made by the households in our sample. We employ multivariate techniques with the goal of identifying the broad relationships present. However, several of the "lessons" learned in the last chapter from reviewing the adjustments made by this group suggest that establishment of such causal relationships is at best a demanding task.

The balance of the chapter consists of four parts. The next section states the highlights of the prior chapter that are especially germane for this analysis. The following section describes the overall analysis strategy, including defining the dependent variables employed and types of models estimated. Presentation of findings follows. And in the final section we offer some conclusions.

LESSONS FROM THE INCIDENCE ANALYSIS

A number of points emerge from the findings of the last chapter that have a direct bearing on the models tested in this chapter. These can be summarized as follows:

Three types of housing adjustments—bringing a roomer or boarder into the home, changing the use of a room, and modifying the dwelling so as to better meet the needs of an impaired person—all occur on a highly discrete basis and households rarely undertake them. The low average incidence, combined with the fact that typically a household will only make one such change over a several year period, suggests that causal modeling may be difficult.

A similar pattern of discrete undertakings also applies to a considerable range of dwelling repair and improvement activity. While many households do make some repairs or improvements each year, the type of actions, their cost, and their number vary sharply for the same household year by year. The degree of discontinuity is greater for elderly households than their more youthful counterparts. Few households were found to neglect repair and improvements year after year.

Regarding the dwellings occupied, these homes were found to exhibit an impressive amount of structural problems (as rated by trained inspectors) at the start of the observation period. But if the evidence on persistency of various dwelling problems which we were able to track over the period is any guide, most of these problems are remedied once they are discovered by their owner-occupants. Very few units show a pattern of problems remaining unattended over several years.

The layouts of the units included in the sample are surprisingly adaptable to families with members with activity limitations. Most have their living space on a single floor. And only about 20% do not have both a bedroom and bath on the first floor. These unit attributes sharply reduce the need for extensive dwelling modifications.

The overall picture of the older households included in this study is definitely one of aging over the observation period, as indicated by reduced working, the increase in the number of single-person households to 35% of the total by the end of the period, and the decline in the share of households that are simple husband-wife households. In addition, all of the information points to there being a great deal of churning in living arrangements and in the number of persons present in a household from year-to-year. This dynamic pattern suggests that there may be considerable opportunity for living arrangements to be modified to provide supportive services without the elderly household having to relocate.

The elderly are seen to have a wide range of contacts outside of the home which presumably stimulate them and which can be a source of assistance when needed, particularly on an episodic basis. Among various sources, those through the church and those with their children are clearly paramount, to judge by regularity and frequency of contact. Importantly, the frequency of contact with children was found to be highly stable over time, despite a good deal of residential mobility on the part of the children. We hypothesized earlier that contact with children may be important for making housing adjustments, both for directly accomplishing them and for providing advice and support. Those lacking such aid may well make fewer adjustments of the type being studied here.

The picture of activity limitations and corresponding supportive services received is very definitely one of episodic problems and responses. While both activity limitations and assistance are highly prevalent each year, there is little incidence of either persisting over a several year period. Apparently those with more serious and persistent problems are unable to remain in their homes. The episodic pattern makes modeling of dwelling modifications and room use changes more difficult, since in effect one has to attempt to identify the episode that caused the family to decide to make the change. In contrast, the onset of a persistent long-term condition could be more readily related to such changes. For this reason it is particularly important to identify those few persons with persistent problems in the analyses.

The information on the economic circumstances of households points to a combination of stability over time for most households and considerable change in the economic ranking of others over the observation period. Such income or wealth changes, especially reductions, could strongly affect the timing of undertaking major dwelling modifications or improvements; or it could cause the family to consider taking in a roomer or boarder.

ANALYSIS STRATEGY

The approach to doing the multivariate econometric analysis has been largely determined by five characteristics of the problem and the structure of the data available for analysis. These characteristics are:

—The dependent variables are all limited, i.e., binary in form, because we have elected to structure the problem in a probabilistic framework.

— The incidence of some of the dependent variables is very low in individual survey data waves; some even have low incidences across waves.

— Conceptually at least, the various housing adjustments can be considered to be jointly determined.

— There are differing numbers of observations over time for some of the independent variables.

— We want to exploit the longitudinal aspects of the data to the maximum degree possible.

Our approach to dealing with each of these factors is discussed seriatim. It should be emphasized at the outset, however, that at points we have decided to employ less than the most sophisticated techniques because of the exploratory nature of some of this analysis and the resource restrictions under which the work was carried out.

Limited Dependent Variables of Low Incidence

The dependent variables in the models we estimated are listed in the first column of Table 5.1. As mentioned earlier, all are in the probability form. Standard multiple regression techniques can be employed in the analysis of limited dependent variables when the mean value of such variables is in the range of 0.3 to 0.7 with only minor adverse consequences. Use of such techniques outside of this range, however, involves considerable loss in the efficiency of the estimates (Maddala, 1983). Almost all of the dependent variables (housing adjustments) in this analysis have incidence rates outside of this "safe" range. For this reason we decided that we wanted to employ logit techniques for all of the final models to be estimated. It turned out, however, that the structure of the models we are estimating is such that it was not possible to obtain reliable estimates using the logit techniques.[1] Consequently, we have used a generalized least squares regression procedure whenever possible to estimate linear probability models that are statistically efficient.[2]

TABLE 5.1

DEPENDENT VARIABLES IN ESTIMATED MODELS OF HOUSING ADJUSTMENTS

Variable	Defined for Adjustments Occurring Over:
1. Probability of dwelling modification being made[a]	Final 2 years of observation period
2. Probability of repairs and improvements being undertaken	
(a) any repair in each year	Each of last 2 years
(b) if repair made, probability that it is above median value[b]	Each of last 2 years
(c) any major repairs made	Any time in last 2 years
(d) no repairs or only small repairs made	Each of last 2 years
(e) no repairs made	Each of last 2 years
3. Probability of boarder present	Full 5-year observation period
4. Probability of room use change	Last 42 months of observation period

a. Population restricted to households with same respondent in survey waves 3-5.
b. Population restricted to households making some repair in last two years. Household must have spent above the median amount, defined separately for elderly and non-elderly households, in both years.

Joint Determination of Housing Adjustments

An operating hypothesis in the analysis is that the various housing adjustments that we have been considering separately are potentially jointly determined. For example, taking in a roomer or boarder may require major investments in the home to assure privacy, etc. Similarly, room use changes may require more alterations than simply changing the furniture, or room use may be changed to accommodate a boarder. It is possible to obtain some sense of the amount of such jointly determined adjustments by studying the number of households that made more than one housing adjustment over the entire observation period. Table 5.2 presents data on this point. The top panel is for nonelderly households, the lower panel for the elderly. It gives the count of the number of households making pairs of adjustments over the approximately five year period (the top row of figures) and over the last

TABLE 5.2

JOINT OCCURRENCE OF HOUSING ADJUSTMENTS
OVER FIVE YEARS AND TWO YEARS
(Number of Occurrences)[a]

	Change in Room Use	Dwelling Modification	Boarder Present
Non-elderly Households			
Dwelling modification	2,35[b] (2,21)[c]		
Boarder present	1,28 (0,10)	0,19 (0,10)	
Major repairs or improvements done	15,122 (3,54)	9,113 (5,51)	2,102 (0,43)
No or only minor repairs done over the period	0,24 (1,38)	0,15 (0,35)	0,8 (0,27)
Elderly Households			
Dwelling modifications	4,62 (1,28)		
Boarder present	1,25 (0,12)	5,55 (1,24)	
Major repairs or improvements done	7,94 (3,41)	20,124 (5,53)	3,87 (0,37)
No or only minor repairs done over the period	2,44 (0,22)	3,56 (0,52)	0,40 (0,15)

a. Total household counts: nonelderly = 138; elderly = 177.
b. Five-year data. First figure is the number of households making both adjustments. The second figure is the sum of the number of households making each of the two separate adjustments.
c. Two-year data.

two years of the period (the second set of figures which are in parentheses). A pair of numbers is shown in each cell of the table: the first is the number of joint occurrences, and the second is the number of households reporting either of the two adjustments involved. With the exception of the joint occurrence of major repairs with changes in room usage and dwelling modifications, there is almost no overlap in households who made different types of adjustments to their units.

These data argue for estimating single equation models for all of the adjustments with the single exception of major repairs and dwelling modifications. While using simultaneous techniques for

these two adjustments is desirable, such estimates are quite complicated when they involve limited dependent variables. We decided,
therefore, to proceed at this time with single equation estimates for
all of the adjustments. We have, however, estimated the dwelling
modification and major repair models with and without the other
variable as an independent variable to obtain a sense of the bias to
the other coefficients that might be introduced by assuming inde-
pendence of these two adjustments.

Varying Observations and Exploiting the Longitudinal Data

As explained previously, the analysis file contains variables for
which we have from one to nine observations (from all five household surveys); those for which we have three observations (waves
3-5); those for which we have only baseline data (neighborhood and
detailed dwelling inspections); and repair data for which we have
nine observations—three from household surveys and six four-
month observations.[3] Additionally, laying out the regression models
has been somewhat complicated by the need to use different observation periods for the dependent variables: for those with very low
incidence rates we have had to use an "any change over the five
year period" format, while for those with a higher incidence in
single years we have been able to focus on changes only over the
last two years. The right hand column in Table 5.1 shows the analysis period used for each set of dependent variables.

The differences in the period for which the dependent variables
are defined has meant taking two somewhat different approaches to
defining the models actually estimated.[4] Both of the approaches
draw from the same set of independent variables, which are listed in
Table 5.3, where an "X" indicates the inclusion of a variable in the
model for the dependent variable listed at the head of the column.[5]
(The independent variables are discussed further below.) Both approaches also have in common that they proceed from quite simple
model formulations to more complex ones. They differ in important
ways, however, in the survey waves from which data are drawn.
We now detail these differences.

TABLE 5.3

INDEPENDENT VARIABLES INCLUDED IN THE MULTIVARIATE ANALYSES

Basic Independent Variables[a]	Dependent Variables: Probability of:			
	Dwelling Modifications	Repairs/ Improvements	Boarders Present	Room Use Change
A. Household Composition				
Set of dummy variables for types of living arrangements	X	X	X	X
Set of dummy variables for change in degree of potential support provided by household	X	X	X	X
B. Activity limitations – each variable defined separately for respondent and spouse if any.				
Weighted sum of limitations[b]	X	X	X	X
Use of special equipment incl. wheelchair	X	X	X	X
Presence of a disabled person in household besides respondent and spouse	X			X
C. Social support interaction				
Contact with children not living at home:				
see one at least weekly	X	X	X	X
talk to one at least weekly	X	X	X	X
Attends church regularly	X	X	X	X

a. Excludes additional variables based on those which record change in status over time.

b. Score = sum over 6 activity limitations (limitation present (0/1)* weight)/3. Weights are for frequency of problem: 3 = all the time; 2 = most of the time; 3 = occasionally.

D. Help with activity of daily living

No. of months meals received	X	X	X X
No. of months attending senior center	X	X	X X
No. of months receiving help with transportation	X	X	X
Assistance variables defined separately for head and spouse			
Longest time any help from outside of home received (months)	X	X	X
Longest time any paid help received	X	X	X
No. of services received from outside of home (10 possible)	X	X	X
No. of services paid for (10 possible)	X	X	X

E. Economic position – dummy variables defining quartiles of:

Income	X	X	X
Net Wealth	X	X	X
Disposable income/total income	X	X	X

F. Dwelling conditions

Problems present at baseline

- unit rated as barely habitable	X		
- unit rated as low quality	X		
- presence of structural problems c	X		
- presence of other exterior problems d	X		
- composite of ongoing problems e			

c. Structural areas included are: roof structure and surface, foundation, exterior walls.

d. Problems include those with gutters and downspouts, exterior stairs and rails, and accumulations of litter and trash.

e. Defined as a count of the presence of the following problems: roof leaks, toilet problems, problems with heat service, problems with electrical service.

TABLE 5.3 (Continued)

INDEPENDENT VARIABLES INCLUDED IN THE MULTIVARIATE ANALYSES

	Dependent Variables: Probability of:			
Basic Independent Variables[a]	Dwelling Modifications	Repairs/ Improvements	Boarders Present	Room Use Change
G. Dwelling configuration - Dummy variables for multi-story units				
- bedroom, no bath on first floor	X			X
- both bedroom and bath on first floor	X			X
H. Neighborhood conditions - dummy variables for:				
- abandoned cars present		X		
- extensive trash & litter present		X		
- industrial uses on block		X		
- street is major artery		X		
- other units on street are substandard		X		
I. Plans to move				
Household says it plans to move	X	X		X
J. Price of repairs - share of repairs done by:				
- head or spouse		X		
- other family members, inside or outside of home		X		
K. "Habit formation" for repairs		X		

First Approach: Dependent Variables
Defined for Two Year Period

As shown in Table 5.1, this group of variables includes the probability of (a) a household making a modification to its unit over this period to facilitate use of the unit by an impaired member; and (b) the persistency and extensiveness of different levels of repair and improvement activity over the period. With the dependent variables defined for the last two years, the principle in the early analysis is for the independent variables to be drawn from data in prior survey waves. In the "simple" models, the independent variables are defined as of household survey wave 3.[6] In addition, dummy (0/1) variables are introduced to indicate changes between waves 1 and 3 in these variables; separate dummy variables are defined for different directions of change, e.g., from less to more income (or another variable for the opposite change) or from a potentially more supportive living arrangement to a less supportive one.

In the "intermediate analysis" additional data are introduced from the same time period as the adjustments. In particular, variables indicating changes in the independent variables between wave 3 and wave 5 are included for some of the independent variables. While this procedure has the advantage of recording changes closer in time to the housing adjustment, it has the disadvantage that the change may have occurred either previous to or after the actual adjustment. If it is afterwards, then the causal ordering is clearly misspecified. To deal with this problem, and to make maximum use of having information on the month in which housing adjustments were made and some changes occurred, we attempted to estimate the "complex" models. These models are the same as the "intermediate ones" except for the variables indicating changes between waves 3 and 5. Two of the dependent variables under analysis here (see Table 5.1), housing modifications and making a major improvement, are defined so that we can distinguish which period an event occurred in.[7] We defined the independent variables indicating changes to have a value of one if (a) there was a change in the independent variable in the period, i.e., between waves 3 and 4 or 4 and 5; and (b) the event of interest (i.e., a housing adjustment) took place in that period *or* a later period. This procedure allowed us to locate changes in the independent variables in time so as not to include those changes occurring after the housing adjustment. Unfortunately, this also led to substantial spurious correlation. Consequently, the results reported do not employ this procedure.[8] Rather those for the intermediate models are presented.

There is one other note on the estimation of these models concerning the population of households employed in the analysis. We observed in Chapter 4 that it was possible for the respondent to differ between survey waves and that such variation can introduce considerable ambiguity into some of the independent variables, especially those dealing with activity limitations and assistance received with activities of daily living. Also, we have hypothesized throughout that activity limitations would be a particularly critical determinant of households modifying their units to accommodate family members with physical impairments. To have the data set best-suited for analyzing the probability of dwelling modifications being made, we use only those observations for which the respondent was the same in the final three survey waves (the waves for which we have activity limitations information). This reduces the number of observations by 35 for the sample of elderly headed households, but we believe that the gain in precision more than offsets the loss in degrees of freedom.

To guard against "respondent change" problems in the other models estimated we have not computed change over time variables applicable to the respondent or spouse (as opposed to the household) when the respondent changed across survey waves. Where the respondent did change, the dummy variables indicating change have been set equal to zero.

Second Approach: Dependent Variable
Defined for Longer Periods

Two types of housing adjustment occurred so infrequently among our sample households that it is necessary, in order to be able to conduct systematic statistical analysis, to define the dependent variable as the probability of the adjustment happening over a more extended time period. These adjustments, and the period covered, are: (a) taking in a roomer or boarder, over 57 months, i.e., the full period between wave 1 and wave 5; and (b) changing the use of a room over the last 42 months of the full period. The different periods are dictated by data availability.

The "simple model" in this case uses the values of the independent variables as of wave 1.[9] The "intermediate model" adds the wave 3 values of these variables as well as wave 3 values for those variables for which wave 1 information is not available. This formulation adds information but some of it may seem to be irrelevant if the adjustment occurred prior to this date. However, these variables may indicate statuses (like activity limitations) that were actual causal factors in the adjustment decision. Excluding them would clearly bias the coefficients of those variables included in the model; but including them also entails problems of interpreting causal relationships. The "complex model" introduces change variables for both the wave 1 (waves 1-5) and wave 3 (waves 3-5) independent variables.

Independent Variables

The foregoing discussion has already covered most of the necessary points about the independent variables that are to be included in the models. As noted earlier, Table 5.3 summarizes the types of variables that were scheduled for inclusion in the models for each of the housing adjustments. The contents of the table essentially review the hypotheses developed in Chapter 2 about the effects of each of these factors on the different adjustments; because of the extensive prior discussion, we only add a couple of comments now. A glance at the entries in the table confirms that most of the independent variables are expected to effect all of the adjustments. The major exception to this rule is that neighborhood conditions, the presence of dwelling deficiencies, "habit formation" for repairs, and proxy variables for the price of repairs (whether they were done by household members or nonresident relatives) are expected only to effect repairs and improvements and not the other adjustments. Similarly, the configuration of the dwelling is expected only to affect modifications being made to the dwelling and the change of the use of a room.

Since the neighborhood variables have not been introduced previously, a brief word about them is in order. The five variables included all indicate the presence of a condition that will likely detract from the value of the property and thus may have the effect of discouraging additional investment in the home.

Another point about the variables included in the various models is that some of the anticipated effects on the housing adjustment under analysis may be quite complex. One example in this regard concerns the effect of the receipt of help with activities of daily living from outside of the home on all of the housing adjustments. Receipt of such help may obviate the need for some adjustments by providing enough assistance to offset the impairment. On the other hand, there may be important indirect effects of the person providing assistance with helping the household organize and implement housing adjustments. Hence, the expected sign of the coefficients of a number of variables in these models is ambiguous a priori, although we may have some hypotheses about which effect should dominate.

A final point is about the inclusion of all of these variables in the estimated models. The number of variables listed in the table is itself large, and we more than double the number through the addition of the dummy variables for the direction of change in many variables over various subperiods within the total time covered by the surveys. It was anticipated that some of the variables would be redundant in that they would be highly correlated, and some of these could be eliminated. It was also expected that many would not be significant—whether because of measurement problems in the variables or because there really is not a significant relationship between the independent variable and the occurrence of a particular housing adjustment. The results presented in the next section are for the models that have emerged after considerable analysis and the pruning of many variables that were consistently insignificant across several specifications of a model. Even with these reductions, however, the models contain a substantial number of variables.

RESULTS

This section reviews the results of the multivariate analysis just outlined. We present the results for each type of housing adjustment separately, beginning with the probability of a boarder being present and ending with the probabilities of various repair and improvement activities. In each case, only the final models are presented and discussed. The general strategy is not to discuss each of the variables included in the models but rather to concentrate on the more salient patterns.

Roomers and Boarders

The final regression models for the probability that a household would have a roomer or boarder present sometime during the five year observation period are given in Table 5.4. Since this table's format is the one used throughout the balance of the chapter, a few comments on its structure and content are in order. The results of a single regression model are presented each for elderly headed and nonelderly headed households. The results for each model comprise two columns of figures. The first contains the regression coefficients, which are interpreted as the change in the probability that the event will occur (e.g., a roomer be present) associated with an incremental change in the independent variable. Because most of the independent variables are dummy variables, the coefficients are interpreted as the change in the probability from the household having a particular condition, e.g., being in the lowest income quartile. The second column contains the significance level at which the coefficient in the first column is different from zero; a figure of .05 means that there is only five chances in 100 that the coefficient is not really different from zero. The summary statistics for the goodness of fit of the models are at the end of the table. An asterisk has been placed next to those coefficients significant at the .15 level or better to help identify them more quickly.

The independent variables are listed in the left-hand stub of the table. With the advantage of having read the previous chapter, the variable labels should be generally self-explanatory. (More information on them is provided in Appendix D.) For those variables drawn from the household survey waves, its name is followed by the survey wave from which it is computed. This is particularly important in these models because some variables only begin with wave 3 and hence changes are computed both from wave 1 to wave 5 and from wave 3 to wave 5.

TABLE 5.4

RESULTS OF MULTIVARIATE ANALYSIS: PROBABILITY OF HAVING A BOARDER DURING FULL OBSERVATION PERIOD

	Elderly-headed Households		Non-elderly-headed Households	
	Coefficient	Significance (P >)[a]	Coefficient	Significance (P >)[a]
Intercept	.084	.41	-.001	.98
Household Type				
Male living alone, W1	.023	.61	-.072	.44
Female living alone, W1	-.051*	.06	.097*	.14
Change to more support, W1-5	.052*	.09	-.027	.46
Change to less support, W1-5	.026	.18	.087*	.02
Economic Position				
Income quartile, W1				
lowest				
second	.012	.70	.014	.78
third	.011	.65	.004	.93
	.002	.93	.015	.72
Income quartile increase, W1-5	-.023	.34	.031	.39
Income quartile decrease, W1-5	.044*	.06	.057*	.13
Rise in share of disposable income, W1-5	.005	.80	-.056*	.10
Decline in share of disposable income, W1-5	.022	.32	.024	.46
Wealth quartile, W1				
lowest				
second	-.019	.51	-.030	.48
third	-.011	.63	-.020	.63
	-.026	.28	-.034	.40
Wealth quartile increase, W1-5	.003	.88	-.038	.29
Wealth quartile decrease, W1-5	-.042*	.02	-.008	.82
Activity Limitations				
Respondent				
Weighted score activity limitations, W3	-.010	.43	-.006	.88
rise in activity limitations, W3-5	-.010	.68	-.036	.59
decline in activity limitations, W3-5	.078*	.01	-.057	.39
Uses special equipment, W3	.109*	.01	-.094	.43
start using special equipment, W3-5	.014	.74	-.151	.28
stop using special equipment, W3-5	-.165*	.01	-.018	.91

Spouse

	Respondent		Spouse	
Weighted score activity limitations, W3			-.075	.23
rise in activity limitations, W3-5			-.117	.35
fall in activity limitations, W3-5			-.228	.23
Uses special equipment, W3			.517*	b

Social Activities/Support

See children weekly, W3	-.049*	.01	-.006	.84
stop seeing children weekly, W3-5	-.012	.66	-.063	.12
start seeing children weekly, W3-5	.028	.36	-.076	.22
Attends church regularly, W3	.008	.63	-.025	.40
stop regular church attendance, W3-5	.034	.22	.178*	.02
start regular church attendance, W3-5	.014	.63	-.012	.80

Assistance Received

Respondent

Received help from outside home, W1	.199*	b		
increase in amount received, W1-5	.044	.29		
decrease in amount received, W1-5	.018	.78		
Number of types help received,[c] W1-5	-.022*	.03	.004	.85
rise in number of help, W3-5	-.031	.52	-.062	.35
fall in number of help, W3-5	-.016	.68	.020	.79

Spouse

Number of types help received,[c] W1-5	.085*	.03	-.091	.52
rise in number of help, W3-5	.049	.49	.350	.25
fall in number of help, W3-5	-.214	b	.099	.73

Summary Statistics

Mean of dependent variable	.050		.032	
R^2	.300		.279	
Adjusted R^2	.113		.094	
F (Significance)	1.61(.03)		1.51(.04)	
d.f.	139		148	

a. Probability that coefficient is not significantly different from zero.
b. Value is less than .005
c. From outside of the home

137

Turning now to the estimated models themselves, it may be best to start with the summary statistics. Both models are statistically fairly weak, as indicated by the small amount of variance in the dependent variable explained by the model and the low level of statistical significance of the overall model, shown by the F-statistic.[10] The general message is that the presence of roomers and boarders evidences little systematic variation. The results may be due to the types of variables included in these models; in addition, however, we should not overlook the problems of temporal specification which arise from modeling change over the entire period with independent variables that may have had changes prior to or after the household taking in a boarder.

The results of the two models (for elderly and nonelderly headed households) are quite different. The model for the elderly has 12 variables that are significant at the 15% level or higher, while that for the nonelderly has half as many. Of these two sets of significant variables, only one variable is both significant and of the same sign in the two models. The balance of this discussion concentrates on the results for the elderly headed households.

Perhaps the most interesting and consistent results are for variables measuring activity limitations and assistance received. Among the elderly respondents, having to use special equipment to get around (as of wave 3) raised the probability of taking in a roomer by about 10%, and a reduction in the use of such equipment over the period significantly lowered the probability.[11] On the other hand, the results indicate that while the intensity of other types of activity limitations was not important as of wave 3, reductions in the level of overall limitations over the balance of the period would increase the likelihood that a household would take in a boarder. This finding might be rationalized in that the impaired person being better able to cope with arranging to take in a boarder. Together the findings point to severe mobility problems pushing households to take in a boarder for assistance, while other activity limitations do not seem to have this effect.

In terms of social support received, the results show that this factor does tend to decrease the likelihood of having roomers or boarders. Elderly who see their children at least weekly are about 5% less likely to have a roomer. On the other hand, the receipt of help from outside the home—from family, friends, or agencies—seems to increase the likelihood of a boarder being present. If respondents were receiving such help in wave 1 (and were still receiving it in wave 3), they were almost 20% more likely to have a boarder. A spouse receiving such help at wave 3 also has the effect of increasing the likelihood of boarders being present. But in contrast, any change in the amount of help received by the respondent or spouse over the period seems to lower the probability. It may be that the variables for the respondent and spouse receiving help in waves 1 and 3, respectively, are indicators of need for some live-in help—possibly because additional assistance from outside the home could not be arranged. Changes in the household's conditions from these baselines may be sufficiently disruptive to plans for other similar households to take in a boarder that the plans are never implemented.

Related to the outside support received, of course, is the household structure. The results show that women living alone are about 5% less likely than multiperson households to take in a boarder. Similarly, a shift in household composition over the period to one potentially providing more support increases the likelihood of boarders being present by about the same amount. These results must be interpreted in light of having controlled for all of the other factors included in the model. Together they imply that having controlled for other sources of help and for activity limitations, that households with more internal support—may be a kind of protection against the stranger—are more likely to take in a boarder.[12] This finding seems important in light of the fact that elderly women living alone are often viewed as the prime candidates for sharing their homes with a roomer or boarder.

Lastly, looking at the economic variables, the pattern is only partially as expected based on our conceptual arguments. The anticipated outcome is that a decrease in income over the period raises the probability of taking in a roomer or boarder by about 4%. Interestingly, a low-income position at the start of the period does not have this type of effect.[13] The unexpected result is that a decrease in net wealth lowers the probability by about the same amount. While one might try to argue that the effects of a change in wealth have longer run implications to which the household adjusts to more gradually and that this would account for this finding, such a rationalization does not hold much attraction for us. We really have no reasonable explanation for this finding.

While the overall models are certainly not very strong, the results do contain some suggestive points. Among the elderly, if the respondent experienced severe mobility limitations and had been receiving help for any extended period from outside the home with routine daily activities, the likelihood of having boarders in the home is sharply higher than for others. Changes in these statuses over the period reduce this likelihood. Multiperson households and men living alone appear to be more willing to take a boarder than an elderly woman living alone; changes in living arrangements to more supportive ones also raise the likelihood of having a boarder. There is also some indication that falling incomes — not low initial incomes — may be a factor pushing households to take in boarders.

Changes in Room Usage

The final models for analyzing changes in the use of rooms within the dwelling that occurred over the last 42 months of the observation period are given in Table 5.5. Looking first at the summary statistics, one sees a sharp increase in the explanatory power and significance of the model for elderly headed households but a decline for the nonelderly, as compared with the results for roomers and boarders. The R-square for the model for the elderly is over 0.9; even without the increased efficiency of the GLS estimator, the R-square was around 0.5. In short, the evidence indicates that room usage change among the elderly is highly systematically related to the types of phenomena included in the estimated model; the opposite is the case for the nonelderly.

The results for the elderly and the nonelderly differ pervasively. Of the 15 significant coefficients for the elderly and eight for the nonelderly, only one is significant and of the same sign in the two models. The balance of the discussion will focus on the results for the elderly headed households.

Again, the key to understanding the results seems to be in the extent of activity limitations and the type and extent of assistance received. Activity limitations on the part of the spouse are especially important in explaining room use changes. If the spouse (in a multiperson household) was using a cane, walker, or wheelchair at wave 3, the likelihood of a room change occurring over the period is 65% higher than otherwise. Increases in the number of activity limitations affecting the spouse over the period also raises the odds of room use changes. Weaker results for respondents may in part indicate the inability of those with serious impairments to live alone. Moreover, if the household has persons other than the respondent or spouse with a physical impairment, the odds also go up. Finally, the more intense the activity limitations of the respondent at wave 3, the greater the odds of a change. Still, the quantitatively largest effects are associated with the spouse.[14] The pattern here is quite clear: room use change is strongly related to activity limitations.

Room use changes are also sensitive to assistance with daily activities provided to the spouse from outside of the household. Such changes are not sensitive to help received by the respondent. The clear pattern is that the greater the volume of such assistance, the lower the likelihood of room use changes. Taken together, the findings on activity limitations and help from outside of the home point to adjustments being much more sensitive to the problems of and help provided to the spouse.

Interestingly, room use changes are clearly and positively associated with the number of months that meals were delivered from outside of the home and transportation services were received. While receipt of such services may signal a higher level of mobility limitations which would cause room changes, it may also be that physical modifications to the unit makes receiving such services easier for the household. Changing the functions of a living and dining room might be done to make the dining area closer to the front of the house. In this regard, it is worth noting that the variables indicating various dwelling configurations were consistently insignificant.

Living arrangements also had some effect on the probability of room changes occurring. Men living alone at the start of the period were about 12% more likely than other household types to under-

TABLE 5.5

RESULTS OF MULTIVARIATE ANALYSIS: PROBABILITY OF CHANGING ROOM USE DURING THE OBSERVATION PERIOD

	Elderly-headed Households		Non-elderly-headed Households	
	Coefficient	Significance (P >)[a]	Coefficient	Significance (P >)[a]
Intercept	.064	.53	.239*	.01
Household Type				
Male living alone, W1	.118*	.08	-.150	.39
Female living alone, W1	.001	.98	-.046	.72
Change to more support, W1-5			-.061	.38
Change to less support, W1-5			-.105	.13
Economic Position				
Income quartile, W1				
lowest	-.078*	.04	-.073	.44
second	-.023	.38	.066	.42
third	.022	.49	.038	.63
Income quartile increase, W1-5	-.036*	.15	-.112*	.08
Income quartile decrease, W1-5	.004	.89	-.096	.16
Rise in share of disposable income, W1-5				
Decline in share of disposable income, W1-5				
Wealth quartile, W1				
lowest	.090*	.03	-.101	.26
second	.001	.98	-.131*	.09
third	.017	.60	-.010	.89
Wealth quartile increase, W1-5	-.029	.54	.077	.27
Wealth quartile decrease, W1-5		.28	.028	.66
Activity Limitations				
Respondent				
Weighted score activity limitations, W3	.022*	.15	.030	.60
Spouse				
Weighted score activity limitations, W3	-.013	.59	.440*	.05
rise in activity limitations, W3-5	.142*	.02	.032	.84
fall in activity limitations, W3-5	.033	.63	-.374*	.15
Uses special equipment, W3	.656*	b		
start using special equipment, W3-5	-.203*	.02		
stop using special equipment, W3-5	-.415	.04		
Others with activity limitations present, W5	.195*	.11		
presence of others begins, W3-5	-.222*	.09		
presence of others stops, W3-5	.170	.25		

Social Activities/Support

Variable	Coef.	Prob.	Coef.	Prob.
Attends church regularly, W3			-.029	.61
stop regular church attendance, W3-5			-.108	.32
start regular church attendance, W3-5			-.012	.88

Assistance Received

Respondent

Variable	Coef.	Prob.	Coef.	Prob.
Received help from outside home, W1	.001	.98	-.002[d]	.28
increase in amount received, W1-5	.024	.68	.206	.66
decrease in amount received, W1-5	-.104	.18	.792*	.05
Number of types help received,[c] W1-5	.004	.79	.071*	.08
rise in number of help, W3-5	-.033	.53	-.362	.44
fall in number of help, W3-5	.084	.21	-.700*	.10

Spouse

Variable	Coef.	Prob.	Coef.	Prob.
Received help from outside home, W1	.114	.62	-.020	.94
increase in amount received, W1-5	-.296*	.03	-.219	.69
decrease in amount received, W1-5	.098	.54		
Number of types help received,[c] W1-5	-.229*	b		
fall in number of help, W3-5	-.225	.21		
Number of months meals received,[c] W3	.010*	b		
start receiving meals, W3-5	-.072	.24		
stop receiving meals, W3-5	-.152	.20		
Number of months transportation services, W3	b	.98		
start receiving, W3-5	-.651*	b		
stop receiving, W3-5	-.020	.80		

Unit Configuration - multifloor units, W3

Variable	Coef.	Prob.	Coef.	Prob.
bedroom on first floor, no bath	.013	.86	.081	.62
both bed and bath on first floor	.032	.36	-.001	.99

Summary Statistics

Mean of dependent variable	.090		.117	
R^2	.984		.165	
Adjusted R^2	.980		-.002	
F (Significance)	206(.0001)		.98(.49)	
d.f.	135		155	

a. Probability that coefficient is not significantly different from zero.
b. Value is less than .005
c. From outside of the home
d. Variable for Wave 3; changes are Waves 3-5

take such changes. Women living alone were not more likely than multiperson households to make room use changes.

The results for the economic variables give rather conflicting signals. Income level at the start of the period does seem to be a factor. Those with the lowest incomes were 8% less likely to undertake adjustments than those in the highest income quartile. On the other hand, the results show those with rising relative incomes over the period are less likely to make such changes. Moreover, households with the lowest wealth levels are more likely to change room use. It is not possible to reconcile these diverse findings easily. Perhaps the most important point is that the effects of all of these economic variables are quantitatively small and are easily swamped by the impact which the presence of activity limitations will have on the probability of changing room usage.

Dwelling Modifications

The final models for the probability of changes being made to the home to accommodate its use by a physically impaired household member are presented in Table 5.6 following the same format used earlier. These models were ultimately estimated using ordinary least squares (OLS) because we encountered the kind of problems discussed earlier when using generalized least squares (GLS) procedures. Both models explain about 40% of the variance in the probability that households will undertake such a modification over the two year observation period — a respectable performance, especially considering that only about 5% of nonelderly households and 10% of elderly households made such adjustments. Both models are also statistically significant under the standard measures.

This model includes an additional variable not present in the models already discussed: whether the household undertook a major improvement (one costing over $1,000) during the period. Also regarding the independent variables it may be worth recalling that for the models for dwelling modifications and repairs, the reference point is wave 3, since the dependent variable is defined for the last two years of the observation period. Two sets of variables measuring change in the independent variables are included in the model: one measuring changes from wave 1 to wave 3 and another measuring changes from wave 3 to wave 5. Finally, the problems of interpreting the wave 3-5 changes should be borne in mind in reviewing the findings. As noted, these problems arise since a change in an independent variable may have occurred after the dwelling modification was made.

The results of the models for elderly and nonelderly households are broadly similar, although there are only two variables that are statistically significant and of the same sign in both models. As expected, a major determinant of the likelihood of modifications is the presence of activity limitations to household members. Activity limitations on the part of the spouse are especially important, although there is some indication that the presence of such limitations for the respondent also has a role. Variables measuring the number and severity of activity limitations and the use of special equipment by the spouse are significant in at least one of the models. [15,16] Typically these variables also have large coefficients. So, for example, in the model for elderly households the fact that the number or severity of limitations increased over the period (waves 3-5), raises the likelihood of a modification being made by 28%.

It is also worth noting that among nonelderly households, the presence in wave 3 of an impaired person other than the respondent or spouse raises the likelihood of a modification by about 15%. Having such a person leave the home during the period also significantly reduces the probability of such an adjustment.

Interestingly, the presence of social support and the receipt of help from outside of the home have rather different effects on the likelihood that the elderly and nonelderly will undertake modifications to their homes. For elderly households, starting to see at least one child once or more per week, having meals brought to their home, and regularly attending a senior center all lower the likelihood that modification will be made. Presumably, these various entities are providing services that offset the need to change the home in some significant way. Similarly, the loss of help from outside of the home raises the probability of modifying the unit. For the nonelderly, however, more support from children or church raises the probability that a modification will be made. But even for

TABLE 5.6

RESULTS OF MODEL OF PROBABILITY OF MAKING DWELLING MODIFICATION OVER LAST TWO YEARS OF THE OBSERVATION PERIOD

	Elderly-headed Households		Non-elderly-headed Households	
	Coefficient	Significance (P >)[a]	Coefficient	Significance (P >)[a]
Intercept	.026	.75		
Household Type				
Male living alone, W3	-.167*	.08		
Female living alone, W3	-.092	.18		
Economic Position, W3				
Income quartile				
lowest	.089	.31	-.004	.92
second	.065	.43	.045	.31
third	.146*	.07	.101*	.02
Wealth quartile				
lowest			-.061	.18
second			-.067*	.13
third			-.052	.22
Activity Limitations				
Respondent				
Weighted score activity limitations, W3	.054*	.15	-.253*	.08
Uses special equipment, W3	.126	.22	.755*	b
start using special equipment, W3-5	.129	.28		
stop using special equipment, W3-5	.042	.81		
Spouse				
Weighted score activity limitations, W3	.023	.72	.088*	.08
rise in activity limitations, W3-5	.275*	.02	-.134	.19
fall in activity limitations, W3-5				
Uses special equipment, W3				
stop using special equipment, W3-5	.234	.38	.522*	b
start using special equipment, W3-5	.119	.40	-.200	.18
Others with activity limitations present, W3	-.288*	.14	.153*	.06
impaired member left, W3-5	-.182	.17	-.176*	.08
Social Activities/Support				
See children weekly, W3	-.084	.16	.058*	.07
stop seeing children weekly, W3-5	-.081	.36		
start seeing children weekly, W3-5	-.283*	.04		
Attends church regularly, W3			.067*	.03

Assistance Received

	Model 1		Model 2	
Respondent				
No. receiving help from outside home, W3	-.003	.91	-.001	.49
No. of types of help received, W3	.197*	.03	-.163*	b
increase in amount received, W3-5	.122	.18	.012	.85
decrease in amount received, W3-5			.474*	b
Spouse				
No. receiving help from outside home, W3	.001	.93	.008	.90
stop receiving help, W3-5	.313	.69		
No. of types of help received, W3	-.048	.92		
increase in amount received, W3-5	-.094	.72		
decrease in amount received, W3-5	-.244	.81		
Household				
No. meal services received, W3	-.006*	.09		
start receiving meals, W3-5	-.193*	.11		
No. attend activity center, W3	-.002*	.02		
No. receive transportation services, W3	.009*	b		
Unit Configuration - multifloor units				
bedroom on first floor, no bath	-.087	.50	.004	.96
both bed and bath on first floor	-.030	.76	-.069*	.15
Intention to Relocate				
Likely to move, W3			-.066	.72
change to "likely," W3-5	-.033	.83	-.220*	.01
change to "not likely," W3-5			.062	.78
Major Improvement to Unit W4-5	.095*	.14	.061*	.10
Summary Statistics				
Mean of dependent variable	.106		.046	
R^2	.404		.467	
Adjusted R^2	.200		.350	
F (Significance)	1.98	(.0039)	3.99	(.0001)
d.f.	105		123	
Estimation technique	OLS		OLS	

a. Probability that coefficient is not significantly different from zero.
b. Value is less than .005
c. From outside of the home

147

this group, help received from outside of the home reduces the probability and a reduction in the receipt of such help sharply increases the likelihood that a modification will be made.

In terms of support within the household, we find that only elderly men living alone are less likely to undertake modifications than those in other living arrangements. Changes in living arrangements, carrying with them more or less potential help within the home, either those for waves 1-3 or those for waves 3-5, were consistently not statistically significant. This pattern is sharply contrary to our expectation and may indicate that modifications are made in fairly stable living environments; if there is some thought that arrangements may change, the modifications are postponed.

Economic position does not play much of a role in determining the likelihood of a modification being made. For both the elderly and nonelderly there is an indication that those in the third income quartile are somewhat more likely than the highest income households (the omitted category in the set of income quartile dummy variables) to make such changes. This is hard to interpret, but might be explained by the highest income group being able to purchase services to compensate for the activity limitations rather than modify their homes. Note, however, that lower income households are no less likely than the highest income group to make modifications. Also, at least as important as these findings is the fact that changes in income position over the period (waves 1-3 and 3-5) were consistently statistically insignificant.

Nor does the configuration of the dwelling have a persistent effect on the modifications made by these households. Only for the nonelderly does the presence of both a bedroom and bathroom on the first floor of a multistory home reduce the likelihood of a modification, and the reduction is about 7%.

Similarly, the stated intention to relocate does not effect the probability that the elderly will undertake modifications. On the other hand, the results indicate that a shift in intention to move among the nonelderly raises the likelihood of modifications. This result is wholly at odds with our conceptual framework, and we discount it as caused by our inability to properly record when the change in attitude toward moving occurred relative to the unit modification.

Lastly, there is a statistically significant relationship between undertaking a modification and making a major improvement to the unit; indeed the two activities are presumably in some cases the same event, but not very often to judge from the small increase probability associated with the household having made a major repair over the period. An examination of models estimated with and without this "major repairs" variable included showed that the coefficients of the other independent variables were not being biased by its inclusion.

We have concentrated on the variables that were found to be statistically important in determining modifications to the dwelling. It is worth stressing in addition that most of the variables measuring changes in the independent variables—either two years previous to or approximately contemporaneous with the modifications being made—were not significant. Changes in living arrangements, economic circumstances, social support, the extent of assistance received from outside of the home, and the likelihood of moving all performed very weakly. These results may be due to the small number of observations available for the estimates, a factor that has clearly limited our statistical work. Alternatively, they may actually be indicating that conditions existing 24 months preceding a household's decision to undertake a dwelling modification are in fact the key in determining whether such an adjustment is made.

Repairs and Improvements

As suggested earlier, the analysis of repairs and improvements differs qualitatively from the other housing adjustments under consideration because they are not readily identifiable one-time events. Rather, households change their level of activity and maintain it over a period of years, with the effects of such shifts only gradually becoming evident. The analysis in this chapter focuses on the extremes: sustained high and low levels of repair and improvement activity. Results for five different models are presented:

- the likelihood that a household undertook any activity in each of the two years of the observations period;
- if it undertook such activity, the likelihood that it made expenditures above the median amount in both years;[17]

— the likelihood that it undertook at least one major improvement
over the two year period;

— the likelihood that it did no or only small (under $100) repairs
in both years; and,

— the likelihood that it undertook no repairs in both years.

The results for the first three of these models, which deal with high
levels of activity, are reported in Table 5.7; the results for low levels of activity are presented in Table 5.8.

These models include several classes of independent variables
not employed in the previous regressions. Added are measures of:
neighborhood conditions; the condition of the structure at the start
of the observation period and indicators of housing problems over
the period; variables indicating who did various repairs (a rough
indicator of the "price" of repairs); and, the average cost of repairs
in previous years (to capture "habit formation" in dwelling upkeep).

We begin by discussing together the results for the *probability of
a household undertaking some repair or improvement activity in
both years* and the *probability that in both years it spent more than
the median amount expended for repairs among sample households*
(Table 5.7, first eight columns). Among the elderly about 69%
made repairs in both years; 80% of the nonelderly are in this group.
Of these households, about 30% in each age category had repair
activity costing more than the median amount in each of the two
years.

The results for these models differ quite sharply from those previously discussed. To begin, the economic position of the household
is clearly a more important determinant here. Especially with regard
to the likelihood of spending more than the median repair cost,
income level at wave 3 was important. Among both the elderly and
the nonelderly, households in the lowest income quartile were about
25% less likely to spend more than the median amount than a
household in the highest income group, after controlling for all
other factors, including who did the work. This differential closes
to about 15% between households in the third and highest income
quartiles. Changes in income position over the full five year observation period do not appear to be important. Nor is the wealth posi-

tion of the household generally a significant determinant. There is the suggestion that higher levels of expenditures among the elderly are considerably more common for those with wealth holdings in the middle of the wealth distribution, but this finding is difficult to interpret. The overall message is that the household's normal income position strongly effect levels of expenditures but it has little impact on whether any repair or improvements are undertaken.

We had anticipated that dwelling conditions would be a clear determinant of repair activity. In fact, for the elderly the results for the variables indicating the presence of major, generally structural, problems with the structures at the start of the full observation period show that those households living in such units are quite unlikely to do much to resolve the problems. Indeed, the presence of such problems at baseline is a very strong predictor of little work being undertaken over the two years for which repairs are being studied. For the nonelderly, baseline conditions had little effect overall, but the one significant coefficient in this group of variables indicates that expenditures would rise in response to such problems being present.

We were also able to include a variable indicating the presence of problems with the basement leaks, heating and other systems at wave 3 as well as changes in the presence of such problems over the period. In general these variables performed poorly, with the significant cases being in the models for expenditures above the median amount; but even here their signs are often counter to what we expect on the basis of our conceptual model. On balance, it appears that most households correct their problems quickly enough that the indicators of minor defects are not good at explaining repair and improvements; on the other hand, among the elderly, those who permit their units to become seriously deficient are unlikely to repair them in the future.

Somewhat surprisingly for both the elderly and the nonelderly, the stated intention to move is associated with more repairs and improvements. This effect is particularly strong for the elderly, with a statement of being likely to move made at wave 3 associated with a 60% increase in the likelihood of making repairs in both of

TABLE 5.7

RESULTS FOR MODELS ESTIMATING THE PROBABILITY OF REPAIR ACTIVITY AND AMOUNT OVER A TWO-YEAR PERIOD

| | Any Repairs in Both Years | | | | If Repairs, Expenditure Above Median | | | | Major Repair in Either Year | | | |
| | Elderly | | Non-elderly | | Elderly | | Non-elderly | | Elderly | | Non-elderly | |
	Coeff.	Signif. (P >)	Coeff.	Signif. (P >)	Coeff.	Signif. (P >)	Coeff.	Signif. (P >)	Coeff.	Signif. (P >)	Coeff.	Signif. (P >)
Intercept	.651*	b	.968*	b	.976*	b	.572*	b	.382*	b	.597	b
Household Type												
Male living alone, W3			.192	.20	.131	.40						
Female living alone, W3			-.026	.82	-.101	.35						
Change in poten. support, W1-3												
more	.280*	.05	-.146*	.10	-.005	.97	-.039	.79				
less	.191*	.06	.036	.69	-.037	.70	.273*	.06				
Change in poten. support, W3-5												
more	.112	.48										
less	.093	.42										
Economic Position												
Income												
Quartile, W3												
- lowest	-.097	.44	-.095	.33	-.301*	.04	-.235*	.07	-.267*	.01	-.052	.44
- second	-.160*	.15	-.078	.37	-.227*	.06	-.215*	.07	-.163*	.05	-.089	.16
- third	-.101	.36	-.011	.89	-.173	.16	-.164*	.14	-.153*	.07	-.043	.50
Change in relat. inc, W1-3												
- more	.006	.94	.007	.92							-.023	.64
- less	.058	.58	-.045	.53							.069	.27
Change in relat. income, W3-5												
- more	-.027	.79	-.088	.25							-.106*	.05
- less	-.113	.29	-.187*	.02							.015	.77
Wealth												
Quartile, W3												
- lowest					.067	.61	-.048	.68			.027	.67
- second					.306*	.01	.015	.90			-.010	.89
- third					.219*	.07	-.130	.23			-.035	.53
Change in wealth, W3-5												
- more									.297*	b		
- less									.032	.69		

Activity Limitations

	Coef.	p	Coef.	p	Coef.	p	Coef.	p	Coef.	p	Coef.	p
Respondent												
Weighted score of limitations, W3	-.083*	.08					-.079	.51	.041	.27	.073	.30
- score rises, W3-5			-.055	.34	.152	.27	-.208	.29	.191*	.04	-.087	.42
- score falls, W3-5					.247	.39	-.284*	.10	-.032	.72	-.132	.18
Uses special equipment, W3	.086	.48	-.076	.64	.745*	b	.126	.76	-.049	.64	-.140	.41
- stopped using, W3-5							-.624	.20	-.088	.59	.273	.30
- started using, W3-5							.173	.60	.236	.24	.109	.51
Spouse												
Weighted score of limitations, W3	.103*	.08			-.010	.80	.250*	.02				
- score rises, W3-5												
- score falls, W3-5												
Uses special equipment, W3	-.388*	.08			-.200	.22	-.402	.27				
- stopped using, W3-5					-.084	.72						
- started using, W3-5												

Social Activity/Support

	Coef.	p	Coef.	p	Coef.	p	Coef.	p	Coef.	p	Coef.	p
See children weekly, W3	.032	.67							-.082	.16		
stopped seeing children wkly, W3-5											.020	.70
started seeing children wkly, W3-5											.019	.86
Attends church regularly, W3	.078	.37							.018	.80		
stopped attending regularly, W3-5									-.230*	.03		
started attending regularly, W3-5									-.026*	.02	.131*	.06

Assistance Received

	Coef.	p	Coef.	p	Coef.	p	Coef.	p	Coef.	p	Coef.	p
Respondent												
Mo. recv. help fm outside home, W3	-.002	.81			.001	.95	-.002	.50			-.026	.24
No. of types of help recvd, W3	.013	.72			-.024	.58	.051	.27			-.031	.76
decline in no., W3-5					-.896*	b					-.057	.48
increase in no., W3-5					-.015	.92						
Spouse												
Mo. recv. help fm outside home, W3	.003	.26					-.223	.18				
No. of types of help recvd, W3	-.016	.92										

a. Probability that coefficient is not significantly different from zero.
b. Value is less than .005.
c. Refers to starting or stopping transportation services.

153

TABLE 5.7 (Continued)

RESULTS FOR MODELS ESTIMATING THE PROBABILITY OF REPAIR ACTIVITY AND SIZE OVER A TWO-YEAR PERIOD

	Any Repairs in Both Years				If Repairs, Expenditure Above Median				Major Repair in Either Year			
	Elderly		Non-elderly		Elderly		Non-elderly		Elderly		Non-elderly	
	Coeff.	Signif. (P >)	Coeff.	Signif. (P >)	Coeff.	Signif. (P >)	Coeff.	Signif. (P >)	Coeff.	Signif. (P >)	Coeff.	Signif. (P >)
Household												
Mo. meal services received, W3	.001	.80			.001	.62	-.055*	.02	b	.51	.042*	b
Mo. transport. svc recvd, W3	.259	.47			-.097c	.67	1.372*	b	-.064	.81	-.391*	.08
Mo. attend activity center, W3	.317*	.12	-.005*	.03	.095c	.56	-.284	.47	.305*	.04	.874*	.01
stopped attending, W3-5												
started attending, W3-5												
Dwelling Configuration												
Bedroom on 1st floor, no bath												
Both bed & bath on 1st floor												
Dwelling Condition												
Overall struct. quality, W1												
barely inhabitable	-.869*	.10							.542	.21	.300	.34
low quality	-.192*	.08			.156	.16			-.069	.46	.091	.23
Critical problems, W1												
foundation, walls, roof	-.030	.77	.133*	.08	-.119	.30	-.079	.48	.014	.86	-.045	.47
other	.069	.55	-.168*	.01	-.081	.42	.197*	.04	-.132*	.14	-.007	.90
Dwelling problems present, W3	.067	.66	-.094*	.10	.214*	.13	-.113	.39	.279*	.04	-.098	.16
Change in dwelling problems, W1-3												
more			.176	.21			-.048	.80	-.272*	.10	-.239*	.06
fewer			.014	.84			.191*	.06	.167*	.04	-.086*	.14
Change in dwelling problems, W3-5												
more	-.112	.38	-.056	.56	-.303*	.15	.049	.73	-.077	.44	.022	.75
fewer	-.095	.65	.049	.68	.031	.78	.303*	.06	-.169	.32	.148*	.11
Neighborhood Conditions, W1												
Abandoned cars	.115	.40	-.416*	b	-.207*	.09	.734*	.03	.034	.75	.623*	.004
House on major artery	.086	.54	-.148	.31	-.186	.21	-.185	.29	.253*	.03	-.078	.31
Substandard houses on block	.033	.84			.164	.19	.328	.15	.098	.46		

In each model cell below, the coefficient is shown first and the probability value (footnote a) in parentheses.

	(1)	(2)	(3)	(4)	(5)	(6)
Neighborhood Conditions, W1						
Abandoned cars	.115 (.40)		-.207* (.09)	.734* (.03)	.034 (.75)	.623* (.004)
House on major artery	.086 (.54)	-.416* (b)	-.186 (.21)	-.185 (.29)	-.253* (.03)	-.078 (.31)
Substandard houses on block	.033 (.84)	-.148 (.31)	-.164 (.19)	.328 (.15)	.098 (.46)	
Intention to Move						
Likely to move, W3	.610* (.05)	.125 (.48)	.064 (.74)	-.357 (.45)	-.302 (.46)	-.030 (.83)
change to "likely," W1-3					1.036* (.04)	
change to "not likely," W1-3		-.444 (.01)			.025 (.86)	
change to "likely," W3-5	.032 (.89)			.482* (.02)	-.257 (.18)	
change to "not likely," W3-5	-1.334* (.02)			.474 (.36)	-.858* (.07)	
Modifications Made to Unit, W4-5	.244* (.05)	.177 (.18)	-.045* (b)	.138 (.44)	.252* (.01)	.145 (.33)
Cost of Repairs						
Avg. share of repairs made by:						
husband, spouse, W4-5			-.106 (.43)		-.199* (.04)	-.054 (.36)
other fam. in/out of home, W4-5			-.154 (.39)		-.406* (.01)	.076 (.64)
Avg. cost of repairs, W2-3 ($1,000)	.058* (.11)	.057 (.36)	.078 (.48)	.023 (.78)		
Summary Statistics						
Mean of dependent variable	.693	.801	.293	.306	.186	.224
R^2	.244	.279	.654	.378	.346	.656
Adjusted R^2	.029	.157	.430	.158	.167	.559
F (significance)	1.13 (.293)	2.28 (.0009)	3.74 (.0001)	1.72 (.0150)	1.93 (.0033)	6.75 (.0001)
Degrees of freedom	137	159	81	110	138	145
Estimation technique	OLS	OLS	GLS	OLS	OLS	GLS

a. Probability that coefficient is not significantly different from zero.
b. Value is less than .005.
c. Refers to starting or stopping transportation services.

155

TABLE 5.8

RESULTS FOR MODELS ESTIMATING THE PROBABILITY OF SMALL OR NO REPAIR ACTIVITY OVER A TWO-YEAR PERIOD

| | Only Small or No Repairs in Two Years | | | | No Repairs In Two Years | | | |
| | Elderly | | Non-elderly | | Elderly | | Non-elderly | |
	Coeff.	Significance (P >)[a]	Coeff.	Significance (P >)[a]	Coeff.	Significance (P >)[a]	Coeff.	Significance (P >)[a]
Intercept	-.010	.92	-.073	.52	.070	.24	-.016	.69
Household Type								
Male living alone, W3	.211*	.11			.043	.55		
Female living alone, W3	.060	.51			-.016	.74		
Change in potential support, W1-3								
more			.019	.81				
less			-.172*	.04				
Economic Position								
Income								
Quartile, W3								
- lowest	.001	.99	.070	.45	.048	.46	-.025	.55
- second	.259*	.01	.147*	.09	.039*	.12	-.008	.82
- third	.183*	.06	-.024	.76	.033	.56	-.035	.34
Change in relative income, W1-3								
- more			.190[c]	.02			-.039	.22
- less			.098[c]	.25			-.032	.32
Change in relative income, W3-5								
- more			-.075	.32			.082*	.01
- less			-.052	.51			.017	.62
Wealth								
Quartile, W3								
- lowest	.137	.20	.033	.70	-.068	.25	.012	.76
- second	.092	.36	.171*	.04	.048	.39	.035	.33
- third	.010	.92	.172*	.03	.066	.24	.048	.17
Activity Limitations								
Respondent								
Weighted score of limitations, W3	-.015	.70	.062	.43	-.001	.94	-.053*	.04
- score rises, W3-5			-.191*	.15				
- score falls, W3-5			.063	.60				

	M1 coef	M1	M2 coef	M2	M3 coef	M3	M4 coef	M4
Uses special equipment, W3	.007	.95	.372*	.12	.053	.39	.313	.01
- stopped using, W3-5	-.141	.42	-.373*	.13			-.320*	.03
- started using, W3-5	-.247	.26	-.342	.28				
Spouse								
Weighted score of limitations, W3-5	-.012	.80	.056	.34	.025	.44	.089*	b
- score rises, W3-5					-.086	.30		
- score falls, W3-5					-.105	.20		
Uses special equipment, W3					.024	.83		
started using, W3-5	-.205	.28	.368*	.15	-.121	.42	-.161	.18
Social Activity/Support								
See children weekly, W3	.053	.45	-.018	.77	-.006	.87	.066*	.02
stopped seeing children weekly, W3-5	.025	.81	-.093	.44			-.067	.22
started seeing children weekly, W3-5	.158	.18	-.126*	.10			-.018	.60
Attends church regularly, W3			.072	.21	-.083*	.05		
Assistance Received								
Respondent								
Mo. received help from outside home, W3	-.001*	.08	-.002	.22	-.001	.23		
Mo. of types of help received, W3	.008	.78			-.022	.20		
Spouse								
Mo. received help from outside home, W3	-.001	.38	.791*	.01	.001	.60		
Mo. of types of help received, W3-5			-.593*	.03	-.124	.16		
increase in no. of help, W3-5					-.007	.71		
decrease in no. of help, W3-5					.104	.56		
Household								
Mo. meal services received, W3	.007*	.06	-.014	.21	.005*	.04		
Mo. transport. services received, W3	-.001	.18	-.001	.85	-.001*	.07		
Mo. attend activity center, W3								
Dwelling Condition								
Overall structural quality, W1	-.349	.48			-.194	.46		
barely inhabitable	.328*	.01			-.131*	.02		
low quality								

---

a. Probability that coefficient is not significantly different from zero.
b. Value is less than .005.
c. For this model change is for Waves 3-5.

TABLE 5.8 (Continued)

RESULTS FOR MODELS ESTIMATING THE PROBABILITY OF SMALL OR NO REPAIR ACTIVITY OVER A TWO-YEAR PERIOD

	Only Small or No Repairs in Two Years				No Repairs in Two Years			
	Elderly		Non-elderly		Elderly		Non-elderly	
	Coeff.	Significance (P >)[a]	Coeff.	Significance (P >)[a]	Coeff.	Significance (P >)[a]	Coeff.	Significance (P >)[a]
Critical problems, W1								
foundation, walls, roof	-.096	.31	-.071	.32	-.034	.50	-.039	.24
other	-.100	.31	-.003	.96	-.047	.40	.017	.34
Dwelling problems present, W3	-.009	.95	.073	.40	-.122*	.10	.002	.92
Change in dwelling problems, W1-3								
more	-.076	.68	-.156	.23				
fewer	-.112	.21	-.002	.98				
Change in dwelling problems, W3-5								
more	-.059	.53	.025	.81	-.019	.76		
fewer	.139	.46	.006	.95	-.344*	b		
Neighborhood Conditions, W1								
Abandoned cars	-.166	.17	.166	.44	-.017	.79	.281*	b
House on major artery	.013	.92	.150*	.11	-.081	.26	.123	b
Substandard houses on block	.041	.77	.067	.64	-.055	.50	.048	.45
Intention to Move								
Likely to move, W3	-.670*	.13	-.154	.35	-.387*	.12	-.029	.86
change to "likely," W1-3	.394	.43			.274	.32		
change to "not likely," W1-3	-.233	.16			-.060	.52		
change to "likely," W3-5							.124*	.07
change to "not likely," W3-5							.010	.96
Modifications Made to Unit, W4-5			-.095	.50			-.030	.64

158

Cost of Repairs

	(1)	(2)	(3)	(4)
Average share of repairs made by:				
husband, spouse, W4-5	.068	.22	.98	.78
other fam. in/out of home, W4-5	.005	.176		
Average cost of repairs, W2-3 ($1,000)	.001	.002	.001	-.008
	.117	.35		
	.97	.53		
	.51			
Summary Statistics				
Mean of dependent variable	.203	.139	.051	.032
R^2	.284	.306	.219	.339
Adjusted R^2	.074	.091	-.003	.211
F (significance)	1.35 (.105)	1.42 (.063)	.98 (.501)	2.66 (.0001)
Degrees of freedom	136	142	137	156
Estimation technique	OLS	OLS	OLS	OLS

a. Probability that coefficient is not significantly different from zero.
b. Value is less than .005.

the next two years. Apparently, plans to move lead to more vigilance in maintaining the unit, even if no move occurs for a couple of years.

In general, activity limitations and receipt of social support and assistance from outside of the home are less important in explaining repairs than they were for the other housing adjustments. Among the elderly there is some indication that activity limitations and use of special equipment by the spouse to get around do reduce the likelihood of repairs being made consistently over time. But this pattern is not very strong. The results for the variables measuring assistance received are also disparate. Several of these variables, which are significant, have the wrong sign—broadly suggesting that ceasing to receive some type of assistance is associated with a major improvement in the person's ability to organize upkeep or the household being able to turn its attention to these tasks rather than the care of the particular person.

Similarly, the results for living arrangements are not strong. The only pattern of any sort seems to be that changes in living arrangements cause some change in the level of maintenance deemed to be "normal," and more or less activity follows. For the elderly it seems that this is typically a higher level, while the pattern is mixed for the nonelderly.[18]

We now turn to the results of the *likelihood that a household undertook a major repair over the period*. As noted, such a repair is defined as one costing over $1,000. About 19% of the elderly and 22% of the nonelderly households in our sample undertook such a major repair sometime over the two year period.

The results for the elderly and the nonelderly are more divergent for these major actions than they were for the models involving persistently high levels of activity just reviewed. Beginning with economic circumstances, the results show that the income level at the start of the "adjustment period" (wave 3) is important in determining the likelihood of such a major expenditure. Moreover, an increase in wealth position over the period seems to increase the probability as well. By contrast, the economic position of the nonelderly makes little difference. This pattern may imply that a sufficient share of these large expenditures, at least for the nonelderly, are for nondiscretionary work—such as replacing a roof or furnace—and that income is not an effective determinant. Alternatively, even the lower income nonelderly may simply be able to afford such expenditures.[19]

Baseline conditions of the dwelling are less important for these major repairs, although there is some indication that those elderly with significant problems at baseline will be less likely to undertake major repairs. (This seems to be reinforced by the result that an increase in problems over waves 1-3 lowers the likelihood of major repairs.) On the other hand, among the elderly the presence of problems in various systems in wave 3 is strongly associated with undertaking major repairs: the presence of such problems raises the probability of a major repair by nearly 30%. Among the nonelderly any change in the presence of problems with the basic systems seems to be associated with a higher probability of a major repair. The seemingly wrong sign (fewer problems results in a greater likelihood) may indicate a shift in preference by the household for a higher standard of repair.

The results for the neighborhood variables are contrary to our expectations, as they indicate that adverse conditions encourage major repairs; and we have no explanation for this result. For the elderly, a statement of being likely to relocate is clearly associated with major repairs being done. This presumably reflects a calculation that the sales price obtained will more than cover the cost of the improvements being made.

Also, only for the elderly, the consistent pattern of household members doing the repairs around the home is associated with a lower likelihood of a major repair being undertaken. On the one hand, this reflects the lower cost of repairs done with contributed labor, which means that the same improvement could be classified as major or less depending on who did the work.[20] On the other hand, it may well signal that if those normally doing the work cannot handle the job, the family is less willing to have it done by a contractor. It is in this sense that these variables act as an indicator of the price of having repairs done.

To some degree we anticipate that major improvements will be associated with making modifications to the dwelling. This expectation is borne out for the elderly but not for the nonelderly. Among the elderly, making a modification to the unit over the two year period raises the probability of having made a major repair by 25%. Since the activity limitations strongly affect dwelling modifications, the result that such limitations, living arrangements, and supportive services do not play much of a direct role in determining major repairs is to be expected. One result worth noting in this area is that starting to attend a neighborhood activity center on a regular basis is strongly associated with undertaking major repairs for both the elderly and the nonelderly. Our only explanation for this phenomenon is that such centers help with referrals to reputable contractors or otherwise help arrange for needed repairs.

At the other end of the spectrum from those households making major repairs or making repairs and improvements that exceed the median value of repairs each year are those *households who undertake only small (under $100) repairs or none whatsoever in two consecutive years*. Few households report not making any repairs in the two year period: 5% of the elderly and 3% of nonelderly households. By contrast, a significant share report only small or no repairs: 20% of the elderly and 14% of nonelderly households.

In general the results of estimating these models (Table 5.8) are quite weak. Indeed, the model for the elderly for the probability of making no repairs is statistically insignificant. For this reason we focus on the results for the other dependent variable, i.e., that for the probability of undertaking only small or no repairs over the period. Even these models, however, are only significant at marginal levels. The overall message here is that lack of repair activity is less systematically related to the kinds of explanatory factors than the other kinds of housing adjustments we have been discussing.

The results for economic position indicate that those in the middle part of the income distribution are more likely to have only limited repair activity than others. Similar results are evident for the nonelderly. Why the poorest households are not less likely is unclear, unless there are systematically households who experienced a dip in income at the time of wave 3 and thus their behavior is like that of higher income households. In terms of dwelling conditions, poor conditions at the start of the observation period are good predictors of being in this group indicating persistent undermaintenance. More recent problems with various systems have little effect, however.

For the elderly, a stated likelihood of relocating is strongly associated with not being in this group. But neighborhood conditions and the "price" of repairs have no effect on the probability of undertaking only small or no repairs.

Interestingly, among the nonelderly the respondent or spouse having activity limitations or using special equipment clearly decreases the likelihood of making few repairs. There is no similar pattern for the elderly. The results for receipt of assistance are weak for both groups, either being insignificant or of the wrong sign in general.

A final observation concerns living arrangements. The results show that elderly men living alone are about 20% more likely to make only limited repairs than those in other living arrangements, including women living alone. This is contrary to our expectations, but it may reflect the importance of others in the households pointing out the need for repairs and helping to overcome a certain amount of inertia in getting repairs done.

CONCLUSIONS

An overwhelming conclusion of this analysis is that the determinants of the adjustments being studied are highly complex. Perhaps the limited number of observations and the low incidence of some of the adjustments combined to limit sharply the fruitfulness of the multivariate analysis. Still, the hints of the intertemporal relationships between the causal factors and the various adjustments found here suggest that it will take a good deal more work before we have a solid grasp on the underlying dynamic processes involved. In this regard, the next appropriate step in this analysis may be to use these same data to examine those households making adjustments as a set of individual case studies. This may be a way to search out common patterns for the next wave of hypothesis development, rather than pursuing further statistical analysis.

To enumerate the principal conclusions for the individual adjustments, it is useful to group the adjustments into two groups: repair and improvements to the dwelling on the one hand, and dwelling modifications, room use changes, and taking in a boarder on the other. Our results indicate that sustained repair and improvement activity over a period as long as two years is driven by the household's economic position, the predisposition to relocate on the part of the household, and undertaking dwelling modifications (which in turn depends on activity limitations and other factors). In contrast, the other adjustments all appear to be determined primarily by the presence of activity limitations (especially as they affect the spouse or partner in a multiperson household); interaction with children living outside of the home and the family's church; the actual assistance received with daily activities from those outside the home; and use of meals-on-wheels, senior centers and the like. Economic position per se is much less important here.

There are a couple of implications for public policy that should be drawn from these findings. One of these concerns programs designed to encourage the elderly to repair and improve their homes, perhaps as a part of broader neighborhood preservation strategies. The findings show income to be definitely important. And, indeed, the provision of cash grants to low-income elderly homeowners in the Experimental Housing Allowance Program resulted in a sharp rise in expenditure levels for maintenance and repairs. But the results also show that the best predictor of low levels of repair activity among the elderly is the presence of significant problems three years before the start of the period over which we studied repair activity. To reach these households — who would be unlikely to be able to bring their homes up to the standards needed to qualify for a housing allowance payment — would require a very different approach, presumably one characterized by intensive outreach activities.[21]

The second area for which these findings may have direct bearing concerns the home matching programs which are being spawned around the country at a very high rate. Such programs typically aim to match someone looking for a low-rent room with elderly homeowners who live in units that contain more space than they need. The prototypical homeowner is conceived to be a woman living alone. Our results suggest that this phenomenon is still quite rare. Moreover, consistent with other studies, we find that matches are of short duration: no one in our sample maintained a boarder (or series of boarders) over the entire observation period. Such churning means that the administrative cost associated with a full year of a shared unit could be quite high, as it would involve multiple matches. Finally, our findings point to elderly women living alone being *less* likely to accept such arrangements, at least as the arrangements have been presented in the past.

The final observation concerns possible public policies that might be designed to promote appropriate room use changes and dwelling modifications where they are needed to better match a home to the needs of a physically impaired person. The short message is that such interventions must be approached very cautiously. Our findings suggest that households have worked out careful arrangements to meet their needs that involve a wide variety of sources. The key to a successful public intervention will be for changes of this type to the dwelling to complement ongoing assistance. This in turn means that mass, formula driven programs will probably not work; they could easily result in a substitution of publicly-funded modifications for family provided services, or add modifications that displace services already provided by agencies. Rather a more tailored approach, involving greater front-end administrative effort is necessary.

NOTES

1. The models had two problems which made use of logit difficult. First, the number of observations on the smaller of the two groups of dependent variables was often quite small, i.e., on the order to 10-20 observations. A general rule of thumb for successful estimates is that the number of independent variables be no greater than one-tenth of the number of observations of the smaller class of the dependent variable. This rule would indicate one or two independent variables in our case. In fact, we wished to include 30 or more variables. Second, nearly all of our independent variables were also binary, i.e., taking only the values of zero or one; and many of them also had few observations with the value one. This meant that there were many cells in the moments matrix containing very small values which caused severe computational problems.

2. The generalized least squares (GLS) procedure overcomes the problem of inefficient estimates that are caused by heteroskedasticity in the error terms of the model by appropriately weighting each observation. (In particular, each observation is weighted by $[\hat{p} \, (1-\hat{p}) \, \exp\text{-}0.5]$, where $\hat{p}$ is the value of the dependent variable predicted by a model estimated without the weighing procedure applied.)

The estimated coefficients are also unbiased. However, GLS is nevertheless inferior to use of logit estimates because the linear function is likely a less close approximation to the underlying relationship than is expressed by the nonlinear two-tailed ogive curve of the logit. Second, with the GLS technique there is no guarantee that values of the dependent variables predicted using the estimated model will be within the zero-one interval; by contrast, logit constrains the estimates so that predictions would be within this interval. (Where we use the GLS procedure we have constrained the predicted values to be in the 0/1 interval.) For more on the problems of linear probability models and this correction, see Goldberger (1965), pp. 231-236; 248-251.

3. The six four-month observations, of course, can be collapsed into two, one-year observations.

4. There is rather sparse literature on the formulation and estimation of models using panel data. Notable exceptions are Heckman (1981), and Campbell and Mutran (1982).

5. Annex D provides a list of the variables included in the table and their corresponding names that were used in the computer analysis. The reader interested in the exact specification on the analytic variables can look them up in the documentation of the analysis file provided in Katsura and Struyk (1985).

6. For variables for which we have only information at the start of the period, their "wave 1" values are used.

7. The other dependent variables defined for repairs and improvements are for the entire two year period, e.g., repairs activity in *both* years. Hence, it is not possible to divide the period into the separate reporting periods.

8. The spurious correlation arose because the independent variable could only take on a value of one if the dependent variable also had a value of one. (The independent variable could also be zero when the dependent variable had a value of one.) An examination of the models estimated using this coding showed the coefficients of these independent variables to be highly significant with values of near one. Inclusion of these variables also strongly affected the values of the coefficients of the other variables in the models.

We had hoped to be able to do somewhat more refined analysis by weighting the independent (dummy) variables indicating change by the number of months between the change in the independent variable and the date when the housing adjustment occurred. We ran into problems interpreting some of the dates reported by households for when the changes in activity limitations and receipt of informal support occurred which prevented us from pursuing this analysis. However, it seems likely that this more precise procedure would have been subject to the same kind of spurious correlation problem that the technique described in the text encountered.

9. We are able to add a few variables for which information was gathered at wave 3, but which included the status of the variable (e.g., activity limitation) at this earlier date.

10. The model for elderly headed households was estimated using GLS. Interestingly, the R-squared actually fell in the GLS estimate as compared to the OLS

estimate, further suggesting the poor specification of the model. The model for nonelderly households reported in the table was estimated using OLS. When we tried to estimate it using GLS, we had serious problems with singularity of the moments matrix. The choice then was either to sharply limit the number of independent variables and use a GLS procedure or keep the larger set of variables and use the less efficient OLS.

11. The results for spouses of these variables were consistently insignificant. Interestingly, in the model for the nonelderly, the use of special equipment is highly significant for the spouse but not for the respondent.

12. The results for nonelderly households are just the opposite from those for the elderly. If the interpretation just given has any validity, the results for the nonelderly may be attributable to the greater self-confidence of these younger women.

13. Variables for total income and the ratio of disposable to total income were highly correlated. We included only variables for total income in most of the models.

14. Somewhat puzzling is the result that changes over waves 3-5 in the use of special equipment by the spouse in either direction lowers the likelihood of room changes. It might be that a reduction in the use of such equipment consistently means that the person is now mobile enough to make room changes not worthwhile, but this explanation does not seem very convincing. Another finding worth recording is that the variables for use of special equipment by the respondent were consistently insignificant.

15. Recall that the sample used in this analysis contains only those households for whom the same person was the respondent in all of the surveys in which activity limitation and assistance questions were asked.

16. For the elderly, the results indicate that a household member beginning to use special equipment over the period lowers the likelihood of a modification being made. We have no ready explanation for this finding unless it is capturing the very rare case in which a person is shifting from being bedridden to being able to move about in a wheelchair. More likely the result is spurious, reflecting the lack of alignment in time between this variable and modifications being made.

17. The median cost figure was defined separately for elderly and nonelderly households for each year.

18. A final observation on the results concerns the variables on the share of repairs made by different persons (see the next to the last set of variables in the table). These variables were excluded from the model for the probability of repairs over two years because they would only have a positive value if there were repairs; hence, including them would have, in effect, been introducing the dependent variable to the right-hand side of the equation. In the model for the household having repairs valued at above the median amount in both years, these variables were insignificant, seemingly indicating that the "price" of different sources of repairs was not important in general. However, as we see later, they were important for the elderly in determining the likelihood of undertaking a major improvement.

19. Note that the income quartiles were defined separately for the elderly and nonelderly. Hence, the lowest income quartiles for the nonelderly has higher incomes than do the lowest income quartile of the elderly.

20. Cost figures exclude the value of contributed labor.

21. For more on such programs, see Struyk (1985).

References

Aquilar, R. & B. Sandelin (1984), "Realized Supply of Owner-Occupied Houses in Sweden," *Scandinavian Housing and Planning Research*, Vol. 1, pp. 197-213.

Blinder, A.S. (1976), "Intergenerational Transfers and Life Cycle Consumption," *American Economic Review*, 66 (May), pp. 87-93.

Branch, L.G. & A.M. Jette (1983), "Elders' Use of Informal Long-Term Care Assistance," *The Gerontologist*, Vol. 23, No. 1, pp. 51-56.

Brody, S.J., S.W. Poulshock & C.F. Masciochhi (1978), "The Family Caring Client: A Major Consideration in the Long-Term Support System," *The Gerontologist*, Vol. 18, No. 6, pp. 556-61.

Brown, Eric S. (1979), "Maintenance and Upgrading Expenditures by Urban Homeowners: Some Survey Findings." Cambridge, MA: Joint Center for Urban Studies of MIT and Harvard University, Working Paper 56.

Brown, H.J. (1975), "Changes in Workplace and Residential Locations," *Journal of the American Institute of Planners*, Vol. 41.

Brown, L.A. & D.B. Longbrake (1969), "On the Implementation of Place Utility and Related Concepts: The Intra-Urban Migration Case," *Behavioral Problems in Geography: A Symposium*, in K.R. Cox & R.C. Golledge (eds.). Evanston, IL: Northwestern University, Studies in Geography No. 17.

Brown, L.A. & E.G. Moore (1970), "The Intra-Urban Migration Process: A Perspective," *Geografiska Annaler*, Series 52B, pp. 1-13.

Campbell, R.T. & E. Mutran (1982), "Analyzing Panel Data in Studies of Aging: Applications of the LISREL Model," *Research on Aging*, Vol. 4, No. 1, pp. 3-41.

Campbell, R.T. & C.M. Hudson (1985), "Synthetic Cohorts from Panel Surveys: An Approach to Studying Rare Events," *Research on Aging*, Vol. 7, no. 1, pp. 81-93.

Cantor, M.H. (1979), "Neighbors and Friends: An Overlooked Resource in the Informal Support System," *Research on Aging*, Vol. 1, No. 4, pp. 434-63.

Chappell, N. (1983), "Informal Support Networks Among the Elderly," *Research on Aging*, Vol. 5, No. 1, pp. 72-100.

Cronin, F. (1980), "Search and Residential Mobility: Part I, Economic Models of Decisions to Search and to Move Among Low Income Households." Washington, DC: The Urban Institute, Working Paper 249-27.

Danzinger, S., J. van der Gaag, E. Smolensky & M. Taussig (1984), "Implications of the Relative Economic Status of the Elderly for Transfer Policy," in H.J. Aaron & G. Burtless (eds.), *Retirement and Economic Behavior*. Washington, DC: The Brookings Institution.

Domenich, Thomas A. & Daniel McFadden (1975), *Urban Travel Demand: A Behavioral Analysis*. New York: North-Holland Publishing Company.

Dumochel, W. & G. Duncan (1977), *Using Sample Weights to Compare Various Linear Regression Models*. Ann Arbor: University of Michigan, Department of Statistics, Technical Report 72.

Follain, J.R. & S. Malpezzi (1980), *Dissecting Houses Valued Rents: Estimates of Hedonic Indices for Thirty-Nine Large SMSAs*. Washington, DC: Urban Institute Paper 249-17.

Fox, A. (1984), "Income Changes At and After Social Security Benefit Receipt: Evidence from the Retirement History Survey," *Social Security Bulletin*, Vol. 47, No. 9, pp. 3-25.

Fredland, D.R. (1974), *Residential Mobility and Home Purchase*. Lexington, MA: D.C. Heath & Company.

Ginsberg, R., J.R. Pack, S. Gayle & M. McConney (1980), *Household Survey: Wave 1 Interim Report*. Philadelphia: University of Pennsylvania Report to Office of Policy Development and Research, U.S. Department of Housing and Urban Development.

Goldberger A.S. (1965), *Econometric Theory*. New York: John Wiley Company.

Goodman, C.C. (1984), "Natural Helping Among Older Adults," *The Gerontologist*, Vol. 24, No. 2, pp. 138-43.

Goodman, J.L. Jr. (1976), "Housing Consumption Equilibrium and Local Residential Mobility," *Environment and Planning*, 8, pp. 855-874.

Goodman, J.L. Jr. (1980), *Urban Residential Mobility: Places, People and Policy*. Washington, DC: The Urban Institute.

Greenberg, J.N. & A. Ginn (1979), "A Multivariate Analysis of the Predictors of Long-Term Care Placement," *Home Health Care Services Quarterly*, Vol. 1, No. 1, pp. 75-99.

Grilichesher, Zvi, B.H. Hull & J.A. Hausman (1977), "Missing Data and Self Solution in Large Panels." Cambridge, MA: Harvard University, Discussion Paper Number 573.

Hanushek, E. & J. Quigley (1978), "The Dynamics of the Housing Market: A Stock Adjustment Model of Housing Consumption," *Land Economics*, Vol. 54, Fall.

Hare, P. (1980), "Rethinking Single Family Zoning," *New England Journal of Human Services*, Summer, pp. 32-35.

Hays, J.A. (1984), "Aging and Family Resources: Availability and Proximity of Kin," *The Gerontologist*, Vol. 24, No. 2, pp. 149-53.

Heckman, J.J. (1981), "Statistical Models for Discrete Panel Data," in G.F. Manski & D. McFadden (eds.), *Structural Analysis of Discrete Data with Econometric Applications*. Cambridge: MIT Press.

Helbers, L. (1979), *Estimated Effects of Increased Income on Homeowner Repair*

Expenditures. Santa Monica: The Rand Corporation, Working Note Draft WN-197-HUD.

Helbers, L. (1978), *Measuring Homeowner Needs for Housing Assistance*. Santa Monica: Rand Corporation, Housing Allowance Supply Experiment Working Note WN-9079-HUD.

Hill, M.S. (1980), "Measuring and Valuing Nonmarket Time Spent in Maintenance of Major Durables and Home Improvements." Ann Arbor: University of Michigan, Institute for Social Research, draft.

Horowitz et al. (1983), "Continuity or Change in Informal Support? The Impact of an Expanded Home Care Program." Paper presented at the 36th Gerontological Society Meetings.

Howe, B., B. Robins & D. Jaffe (1984), *Evaluation of the Homeshare Program*. Milwaukee: Medical College of Wisconsin, Milwaukee Long-Term Care Gerontology Center.

Ingram, Gregory K. & Oron, Yitzhak (1977), "The Behavior of Housing Producers," in *Residential Location and Urban Housing Markets*, Gregory K. Ingram (ed.), New York: National Bureau of Economic Research.

Jacobs, B. (1982), *An Overview of the National Potential for Home Equity Conversion into Income for the Elderly*. Rochester, NY: University of Rochester, Public Policy Analysis Program, Discussion Paper 8205.

Johnson, C.L. & D.J. Catalano (1983), "A Longitudinal Study of Family Supports to the Impaired Elderly," *The Gerontologist*, Vol. 23, No. 6, pp. 612-18.

Kain, J.F. & J.M. Quigley (1975), *Housing Markets and Racial Discrimination*. New York: Columbia University Press.

Kalton, G. (1981), *Compensating for Missing Survey Data*. Ann Arbor: University of Michigan, Institute for Social Research.

Katsura, H. & R. Struyk (1985), *Documentation of the In-Place Housing Adjustment Analysis File*. Washington, DC: The Urban Institute, Report 3166-04.

Koken, J.A. (1983), "Old But Not Alone: Informal Social Supports Among the Elderly by Marital Status and Sex," *The Gerontologist*, Vol. 23, No. 1, pp. 57-63.

Koyck, L. (1954), *Distributed Lags and Investment Analysis*. Amsterdam: North-Holland Publishing Company.

Lawton, M.P. (1981), "An Ecological View of Living Arrangements," *The Gerontologist*, Vol. 21, pp. 59-66.

Lawton, M.P. (1983), "Environment and Other Determinants of the Well-Being in the Aged," *The Gerontologist*, Vol. 23, pp. 349-57.

Lawton, M.P., M. Moss & R. Kleban (1984), "Marital Status, Living Arrangements, and the Well-Being of Older People," *Research on Aging*, Vol. 6, No. 3, pp. 323-45.

MacMillan, J. (1980), Mobility in the Housing Allowance Demand Experiment. Cambridge: Abt Associates.

Maddala, G.S. (1983), *Limited-Dependent and Qualitative Variables in Econometrics*. Cambridge: Cambridge University Press.

Manton, K.G. & B.J. Soldo (1985), "Dynamics of Health Changes in the Oldest Old," *Milbank Memorial Fund Quarterly/Health and Society*, Vol. 63, No. 2, pp. 206-85.

Mayer, N.S. (1981), "Grants, Loans, and Housing Repair for the Elderly," *American Planning Association Journal*, January, pp. 25-34.

McConnell, S. & C.E. Usher (1980), *Intergenerational Housesharing*. Los Angeles: Ethel Percy Andrus Gerontology Center, University of Southern California.

Mendelsohn (1977), "Empirical Evidence on Home Improvements," *Journal of Urban Economics* (October), pp. 457-68.

Moon, M. (1977), *The Measurement of Economic Welfare: Its Application to the Aged Poor*. New York: Academic Press.

Moore, E.G. (1972), *Residential Mobility in the City*. Washington, DC: Association of American Geographers.

Mundinger, M.O. (1983), *The House Care Controversy*. Rockville, MD: Aspen Systems Corporation.

Murray, P. (1979), *Shared Homes: A Housing Option for Older People*. Washington, DC: International Center for Social Gerontology.

Myers, D. (1984), "Turnover and Filtering of Post War Single-Family Housing," *American Planning Association Journal*, Summer, pp. 352-58.

Nerlove, M. (1958), *Distributed Lags and Demand Analysis*, Washington, DC: U.S. Department of Agriculture. Handbook 141.

Newman, S. (1979), "Exploring Housing Adjustments of Older People: The HUD-HEW Longitudinal Study." Washington, DC: U.S. Department of Housing and Urban Development, Paper presented at the National Institute on Aging Conference on "Demographic and Health Information for Aging Research: Resources and Needs."

Newman, S. (1985), "Housing and Long-Term Care: The Suitability of the Elderly's Housing to the Provision of In-Home Services," *The Gerontologist*, Vol. 25, No. 1, pp. 35-40.

Ozanne, L. & R. Struyk (1976), *Housing from the Existing Stock: Comparative Economic Analyses of Owner-Occupants and Renters*. Washington, DC: The Urban Institute.

Palmer, J.L. & B.B. Torrey (1984), "Health Care Financing and Pension Programs," in G.B. Mills & J.L. Palmer (eds.), *Federal Budget Policy in the 1980s*. Washington, DC: The Urban Institute Press, pp. 121-64.

Pritchard, D.C. (1983), "The Art of Matchmaking: A Case Study in Shared Housing," *The Gerontologist*, Vol. 23, No. 2, pp. 174-179.

Quigley, J.M. & D.H. Weinberg (1977), "Intra-Urban Residential Mobility: A Review and Synthesis," *International Economic Review*, Fall, Vol. No. 18, pp. 41-66.

Reece, D., T. Walz & H. Hageboeck (1983), "Intergenerational Care Providers of Non-Institutionalized Frail Elderly: Characteristics and Consequences," *Journal of Gerontological Social Work*, Vol. 5, No. 3, pp. 21-34.

Reschovsky, J.D. (1983), *Housing Consumption of the Elderly: A New Approach to the Question of Adequacy.* Lansing: Madison College, Michigan State University, Paper presented at Fifth Annual Research Conference of the Association for Public Policy Analysis and Management.

Ridley, J.C., C.A. Bachrach & D. Dawson (1979), "Recall and Reliability of Interview Data from Older Women," *Journal of Gerontology*, Vol. 34, pp. 99-105.

Rossi, P.H. (1955), *Why Families Move.* New York City: The Free Press.

Sangl, G. (1983), "The Family Support System of the Elderly," in R. Vogel & H. Palmer (eds.), *Long-term Care.* Washington, DC: Health Care Finance Administration, pp. 307-336.

Schneider, W., K. Stahl & R. Struyk (1985), "Residential Mobility," in K. Stahl & R. Struyk (eds.), *U.S. and West German Housing Markets.* Washington, DC: The Urban Institute Press.

Schreter, C. (1983), "Shared Housing: Discovering the Value of Living with Non-relatives." Baltimore: unpublished.

Schwartz, S., S. Danzinger & E. Smolensky (1984), "The Choice of Living Arrangements by the Elderly," in H.J. Aaron & G. Burtless (eds.), *Retirement and Economic Behavior.* Washington, DC: The Brookings Institution.

Select Committee on Aging, U.S. House of Representatives (1982), *Shared Housing Hearing, November 17, 1981.* Washington, DC: U.S. Government Printing Office, Committee Publication 97-321.

Soldo, B. (1982), "Supply of Informal Care Services: Variations and Effects on Service Utilization Patterns." Washington, DC: Urban Institute Paper 1466-16.

Soldo, B.J. (1983), *A National Perspective on the Home Care Population.* Washington, DC: Georgetown University, Center for Population Research, CPR 83-004.

Soldo, B.J. (1983a), *In-Home Services for the Dependent Elderly: Determinants of Current Use and Implications for Future Demand.* Washington, DC: Center for Population Research, Georgetown University.

Soldo, B.J. & K.G. Manton (1985), "Health Status and Services Needs of the Oldest Old," *Milbank Memorial Fund Quarterly/Health and Society*, Vol. 63, No. 2, pp. 286-318.

Speare, A. Jr. (1970), "Home Ownership, Life-Cycle Stage, and Residential Mobility," *Demography*, Vol. 7, pp. 449-458.

Speare, A. Jr., S. Goldstein & W.H. Frey (1974), *Residential Mobility, Migration, and Metropolitan Change.* Cambridge, MA: Ballinger Publishing Company.

Stoller, E.P. & L.L. Earl (1983), "Help with Activities of Everyday Life: Sources of Support for the Noninstitutionalized Elderly," *The Gerontologist*, Vol. 23, No. 1, pp. 64-70.

Straszheim, M.J. (1975), *An Econometric Analysis of the Urban Housing Market*, New York: Columbia University Press.

Struyk, R. (1976), *Urban Homeownership: The Economic Determinants.* Cambridge: Lexington Books, D.C. Heath.

Struyk, R. (1980), "Housing Adjustments of Relocating Elderly Households," *The Gerontologist*, Vol. 20, pp. 45-55.

Struyk, R. (1980a), *A New System for Public Housing*. Washington, DC: The Urban Institute.

Struyk, R. (1981), "The Changing Housing and Physical Environment of the Elderly: A Look at the Year 2000," in S. Kiesler, J.N. Morgan & V.K. Oppenheimer (eds.), *Aging: Social Change*. New York: Academic Press.

Struyk, R. (1982), *In-Place Housing Adjustments of the Elderly: Data Acquisition and Sample*. Washington, DC: Urban Institute Paper 3166-01.

Struyk, R. (1982), "The Demand for Specially Adapted Housing by Elderly Headed Households." Washington, DC: The Urban Institute Project Report 3014-01.

Struyk, R. (1985), "Future Housing Assistance Policy for the Elderly," *The Gerontologist*, Vol. 25, No. 1, pp. 41-46.

Struyk, R. & B. Soldo (1980), *Improving the Elderly's Housing*. Cambridge, MA: Ballinger Publishing Company.

Struyk, R. & M. Turner (1984), "Changes in the Housing Situation of the Elderly: 1974-1979," *Journal of Housing for the Elderly*, Vol. 2, No. 1, pp. 3-20.

Struyk, R. & J. Zais (1982), "Providing Special Dwelling Features for the Elderly with Health and Mobility Problems." Washington, DC: The Urban Institute.

Sussman, M.B. (1979), *Social and Economic Supports and Family Environments for the Elderly*. Washington, DC: Report to the Administration on Aging, processed.

Sweeney, J.L. (1974), "Housing Unit Maintenance and Mode of Tenure," *Journal of Economic Theory*, pp. 111-38.

Thomas, S. (1983), "The Significance of Housing as a Resource," in R. Vogel & H. Palmer (eds.), *Long-Term Care*. Washington, DC: Health Care Financing Administration, pp. 391-414.

U.S. Department of Energy, Energy Information Agency (1980), *Characteristics of the Housing Stock and Households: 1978*. Washington, DC: U.S. Government Printing Office, DOE/EIA-0207/2.

University of Pennsylvania (1980), *Baseline Report on Twenty Study Areas*. Philadelphia: Report to Office of Policy Development and Research, U.S. Department of Housing and Urban Development.

Verbrugge, L.M. (1979), "Marital Status and Health," *Journal of Marriage and the Family*, Vol. 41, pp. 267-85.

Weissert, W. & W. Scanlon (1983), "Determinants of Institutionalization of the Aged." Washington, DC: Urban Institute Paper 1466-21, revised.

Wolf, D.A. (1983), *Kinship and Living Arrangements of Older Americans*. Washington, DC: Urban Institute Project Report.

Appendixes

APPENDIX A
THE REPRESENTATIVENESS OF THE
NIA SAMPLE

The sample of households included in this analysis was drawn for purposes other than representing the population of urban households*. In particular, the households were drawn from a three-stage procedure designed to yield a sample useful for analyzing the neighborhood-level impacts of the Community Development Block Grant (CDBG) program. In the first stage, nine cities with populations of over 100,000 were chosen on a purposeful basis to capture the range of strategies in use of CDBG funds, city sizes, and regions of the country. In the second stage, two or three neighborhoods (of about 25 continuous blocks each) were selected in each city on the basis of the use of CDBG funds in them. In the third stage, about 100 households in each neighborhood were randomly sampled.

The current analysis employs data on owner-occupant households surviving the two-survey waves of households conducted under the CDBG study in a total of 14 neighborhoods in seven cities. (Two cities were dropped because of small sample sizes of homeowners.) From the general way in which the sample of households for the present study was assembled, there is every reason to doubt that the sample is generally representative of homeowner populations in urban areas.

---

*Anne Simpson provided able assistance in preparing the calculations presented here.

The purpose of the analysis reported below is to examine the sample used in this study in two ways:

1. Compare the attributes of households in the present sample with those of homeowners living in the central cities of SMSAs throughout the United States.
2. Compare the attributes of the neighborhoods in which the sample households live with those of central city neighborhoods generally.

The characteristics of the neighborhoods are important because they can affect housing investment behavior—a central interest of the analysis in the main study.

Three sets of data are employed in this work. For the neighborhood comparisons, all data are from census tract statistics for 1980. In essence, the weighted average of selected attributes of the tracts in which sample households are located are compared with the average values for all tracts in the central cities of SMSAs.[1] The comparison of household attributes involves two data sets. First, attributes for the households included in this analysis were computed using data for those households for whom full data were available at the end of the first two survey waves.[2] The comparison data—for all households in central cities in SMSAs—are from the March, 1981 Current Population Survey (CPS). (The second wave of the CDBG survey was conducted in February-March 1981.)

Table A.1 displays some tabulations comparing the attributes of CPS households with those of households in our sample. Shown is the distribution of households by age and by income, each stratified by the age of head of household. The upper number in each cell is for the CPS households and the lower one (in parentheses) is for the "study sample." Application of a chi-square test shows that the households in the two samples differ significantly from each other in terms of age distribution and incomes.

The last row of data in Panel A shows the distribution of the sample across three age categories. In the study sample, almost half of the households are headed by someone over 60, while in the CPS the comparable figure is about one-third. The overall distributions of households among the three household types between the two

TABLE A.1

COMPARISON OF SAMPLE OF HOUSEHOLDS IN PRESENT ANALYSIS
WITH SAMPLE OF THE CPS

A.   Percentage distribution of household types
within age categories

| | Age of Household Head | | | All Households |
	under 45	45-49	60+	
Household Type				
couple	65[a] (68)[b]	68 (70)	52 (50)	61 (60)
individual living alone	14 (8)	15 (12)	36 (30)	22 (20)
other	20 (24)	16 (18)	12 (20)	16 (20)
percentage of all households in age group	37 (21)	28 (29)	34 (49)	

B.   Percentage distribution of households by income
within age categories

Income	under 45	45-49	60+	All Households
under $5,000	5 (6)	6 (9)	19 (38)	10 (22)
$5,000-12,999	15 (30)	15 (36)	35 (52)	22 (42)
$13,000-20,999	24 (34)	19 (22)	19 (6)	21 (17)
$21,000-33,999	36 (27)	28 (28)	16 (3)	26 (16)
$34,000 or over	21 (7)	32 (4)	11 (--)	21 (3)

a.   Data from Current Population Survey (CPS); calculated from users tape.
b.   Data from sample for this study; computed for sample at end of wave 2.

samples (last column, Panel A) are statistically equivalent. Within each age category there is somewhat less similarity in the distributions among household types, but the divergence is still fairly modest.

The incomes of the households in the study sample are significantly lower than those in the CPS sample (Panel B). This pattern
holds across all three age categories, although it is most pronounced
for the elderly.

Turning now to the comparison of the neighborhoods in which
study sample households reside and the "average" neighborhood in
America's central cities, the results are given in Table A.2. The
table presents the mean values for six neighborhood characteristics
for the two groups of areas. The attributes describe the housing
stock (tenure, lack of complete plumbing, overall vacancy rate) and
the families living there (percentage headed by a black, a person
over age 65, or a woman with children under 18). We have not used
income, house value, or rent data because of the regional price variations embodied in these data which would bias the comparisons.
Finally the table includes an indication of those characteristics
which were found to differ significantly between the "sample
neighborhoods" and all central cities according to a t-test.[3]

TABLE A.2

COMPARISON OF NEIGHBORHOOD ATTRIBUTES BETWEEN AREAS IN WHICH
SAMPLE HOUSEHOLDS LIVE AND ALL CENTRAL CITIES[a]

	All Central Cities	15 Sample Neighborhood
Percent of households headed by a black	23[b]	42[b]
Percent of households headed by someone 65 or older	12	13
Percent of occupied units owner-occupied	49	57
Percent of dwelling lacking full plumbing	2	3
Percent of households headed by female with children under 18	13[b]	26[b]
Overall vacancy rate (percent)	7	8

a. Data from 1980 census tract statistics.
b. Sample neighborhoods differ from all central cities at the .05
level of significance.

The tests show that the two groups of areas are essentially the same with respect to four of the six attributes. They differ in that the sample neighborhoods have a substantially greater percentage of households headed by a black (42 vs. 23%) and households headed by a woman with minor children (26 vs. 13%). These comparisons of the means mask a good deal of divergence between the sample neighborhoods and the "average" characteristics of the cities in which they are located (Table 3.1). Interestingly, however, the greatest difference are in the two characteristics found to differ more generally: race and young female households.

The overall conclusion of this analysis is that the households included in the sample for this study differ significantly from the population of households who are homeowners residing in the central cities of SMSAs. On the other hand, they reside in neighborhoods that are broadly similar to the "average" central city neighborhood, although there are some important differences.

APPENDIX B
OVERVIEW OF IMPUTATION PROCEDURES

This appendix gives an overview of the procedures used to impute values for those variables with missing values.[4] Although there was a large number of missing values, it is important to recognize that the majority of variables had only a few missing values.[5] In addition, in some instances, consistency checks revealed that "missing" values were the result of cleaning errors that often involved the incorrect coding of not applicable responses. When this occurred, no information was lost by the imputation procedure. As is typical with many surveys, most missing values were generated by the more sensitive questions dealing with a household's financial status. Date values — especially those referring to the month in which some event occurred — were also missing relatively frequently. When assessing the quality of the data, it is important to take into consideration all of these factors.

Many of the imputation procedures adopt a similar approach. Most involve the use of information obtained from another survey wave where nonmissing values from other waves are substituted for missing values. For example, if the response to the question regarding the race of the respondent was missing in wave 3, then the response to the same question in wave 4 was substituted for the missing value in wave 3.

When the substitution technique described above was impossible, produced results inconsistent with other values, or was unreasonable on theoretical grounds, a random procedure was employed. Random imputations were performed by dividing all households within a wave into groups based on characteristics believed to be related to a household's response to a given question. A household was eligible to be a "donor" to a household missing a value (i.e., a "seeker" household) if it fell into the same group or "cell," and if it possessed a legitimate (i.e., nonmissing) response. Values from randomly-selected donors from within the appropriate cell were used to fill missing responses. In general, a seeker household tried to take as much information as possible from a single donor for any given question. If a single donor did not satisfy all missing responses, then additional donors were selected until the requirements of the seeker household were satisfied.

Sometimes a set of criteria failed to produce a suitable donor. When this occurred, the donor pool was expanded either by adopting a simpler set of criteria to define the cells or by including observations from other waves that met the original criteria. It is important to recognize that situations requiring these particular procedures were seldom encountered, and usually involved only a few observations.

In a few instances, regression models were developed and used to estimate values. Once they were generated for a single wave, these imputed values became eligible to be passed to other waves.

Waves 3 through 5 of the household surveys were approached somewhat differently than waves 1 and 2. Because of time constraints, most of the imputations for waves 1 and 2 were completed before those for waves 3 through 5 were completed. The imputations performed for waves 1 and 2 made somewhat greater use of random procedures. This slight difference in methodology, however, does not pose a major consistency problem between waves 1 and 2 and waves 3 through 5 since the questionnaires were different for many areas; only a moderate number of questions were asked during all five in-person interviews. Most of these questions deal with household composition, income, assets, and debts. In general, an attempt was made to make waves 1 and 2 consistent with each other and waves 3 through 5 consistent with each other. For example, when obtaining values for wave 3 from other waves, waves 4 and 5 would be examined for applicable values before waves 1 and 2. Similarly, when searching for a value for wave 2, wave 1 would be examined before any of the other waves. For waves 3 through 5, the following search sequence was followed: when seeking a value for wave 3, check wave 4 before wave 5; when seeking a value for wave 4, check wave 3 before wave 5; and when seeking a value for wave 5, check wave 4 before wave 3.

APPENDIX C

SHIFTS OF HOUSEHOLDS BETWEEN REPAIR ACTIVITY CATEGORIES OVER TIME[a]
(number of households)

	Non-elderly Headed Households					Elderly Headed Households				
	No repairs	Q1	Q2	Q3	Q4	No repairs	Q1	Q2	Q3	Q4
I. Total Number of Repairs										
	Between Surveys 2 and 3					Between Surveys 2 and 3				
Between Waves 1 and 2										
No Repairs	5	10	2	8	3	15	10	13	3	1
Q1	13	26	9	5	8	5	10	8	9	4
Q2	2	11	2	6	6	12	5	5	6	7
Q3	2	9	5	6	11	9	11	3	10	5
Q4	4	12	3	8	11	4	4	2	5	11
II. Cost of Repairs										
	Between Surveys 2 and 3					Between Surveys 2 and 3				
Activity Between Waves 1 and 2										
No Repairs	9	6	6	3	2	15	10	13	7	5
Q1	8	10	9	9	4	9	7	4	5	7
Q2	5	10	10	7	9	7	9	3	10	3
Q3	4	6	6	12	12	6	4	6	8	8
Q4	2	8	10	9	11	5	4	8	4	10

a. Households are classified first into those having any activity and no activity. Those with activity are divided in approximate quartiles.

b. Quartile 1 is the lowest level of activity.

TOTAL INCOME POSITION VS. NET WEALTH AND DISPOSABLE INCOME,
AS OF FOURTH SURVEY WAVE[a]
(percents)

Total Income/Quartile	Non-elderly Headed Households				Elderly Headed Households			
	Q1[b]	Q2	Q3	Q4	Q1	Q2	Q3	Q4
A. Net Wealth								
Q1	32	34	26	8	36	39	20	5
Q2	27	25	32	16	27	22	31	20
Q3	34	26	17	23	15	21	28	36
Q4	11	11	26	52	19	23	16	42
B. Disposable Income								
Q1	90	10	-	-	91	9	-	-
Q2	5	86	9	-	8	76	16	-
Q3	-	8	80	11	-	3	87	10
Q4	-	-	11	89	-	2	5	83

a. Rows sum to 100 percent.
b. Quartiles defined separately for non-elderly and elderly headed households for each survey wave. Q1 is lowest income or wealth group.

APPENDIX C (continued)

SURVEY TO SURVEY CHANGES IN REPAIR ACTIVITY

	Non-elderly Headed Households		Elderly Headed Households	
	In same group[a]	Shift 2+ position[b]	In same group	Shift 2+ positions
Number of Repairs				
W1-W2	27	34	26	42
W2-W3	29	34	29	45
W3-W4	25	32	30	32
W4-W5	34	24	33	26
Cost of Repairs				
W1-W2	24	40	24	42
W2-W3	28	36	29	40
W3-W4	34	34	32	35
W4-W5	25	34	29	40

a. Five groups are defined: no repairs and 4 quartiles (approximate) for those with repairs.
b. Households shifts between waves, for example, from Q1 to Q3 or Q4 or from Q2 to no activity.

APPENDIX C (continued)

DISTRIBUTION OF THE RATIO OF DISPOSABLE TO TOTAL INCOME
BY AGE OF HOUSEHOLD HEAD[a]
(percents)

Ratio Value	Age of Head of Household	
	Non-elderly	Elderly
< .1	2	2
.1-.2	-	1
.2-.3	1	2
.3-.4	2	3
.4-.5	4	4
.5-.6	7	7
.6-.7	13	15
.7-.8	24	26
.8-.9	29	32
.9-1.0	18	7

a. Data from household survey wave 3.

APPENDIX D

This appendix is a reference guide for the variables used in the multivariate analyses presented in the main text of this report. The tables in Chapter 5 use descriptive labels to describe variables; this section provides the names of the variables on the analysis file that correspond to these labels. Anyone interested in the exact specification of the analytic variables can refer to the documentation of the analysis file provided in Katsura and Struyk (1985).

In many instances, new variables were created from the basic analytic variables. Most of these are "change" variables indicating whether the value of a variable increased or decreased over some time period. Changes are usually represented by two dummy variables — one for each direction of change — where each takes on a value of one of a change occurred, zero otherwise. Note that these new variables were not kept for the analysis file.

The descriptions that follow are grouped into several classes of variables. Within each variable group, descriptive labels from the text are matched with corresponding variables from the analysis file. For new variables, brief descriptions of how the analytic variables were recoded are given.

APPENDIX D: TABLE 1

DESCRIPTIVE LABELS	CORRESPONDING ANALYTIC VARIABLES	RECODING
Household Type		
Male living alone, W3	HHTYP3	If HHTYP3=1 then dummy=1.
Female living alone, W3	HHTYP3	If HHTYP3=2 then dummy=1.
Change in potential support		
- more, W1-3	HHTYP1, HHTYP3	Recoded into a dummy using the same support change rules as SUP14, SUP24, SUP34, and SUP44.
- less, W1-3	HHTYP1, HHTYP3	If HHTYP1≠HHTYP3 and support did not increase then dummy=1.
- more, W3-5	HHTYP3, HHTYP5	Recoded into a dummy using the same support change rules as SUP14, SUP24, SUP34, and SUP44.
- less, W3-5	HHTYP3, HHTYP5	If HHTYP3≠HHTYP5 and support did not increase then dummy=1.
Economic Position		
Income Quartile, W3	CTOTY	Recoded into quartiles.[a]
Change in relative income		
- more, W1-3	ATOTY, CTOTY	Recoded into quartiles;[a] if income increased then dummy=1.
- less, W1-3	ATOTY, CTOTY	Recoded into quartiles;[a] if income decreased then dummy=1.
- more, W3-5	CTOTY, ETOTY	Recoded into quartiles;[a] if income increased then dummy=1.
- less, W3-5	CTOTY, ETOTY	Recoded into quartiles;[a] if income decreased then dummy=1.

Wealth Quartile, W3	CNTWLTH	Recoded into quartiles.[a]
Change in wealth		
- more, W3-5	CNTWLTH, ENTWLTH	Recoded into quartiles;[a] if wealth increased then dummy=1.
- less, W3-5	CNTWLTH, ENTWLTH	Recoded into quartiles;[a] if wealth decreased then dummy=1.

Assistance Received

Respondent

Mo. received help from outside home, W3	CRTANY	
No. of types of help received, W3	CRVAR54	
- decrease in no., W3-5	CRVAR54, ERVAR54	If CRVAR54 > ERVAR54 then dummy=1.
- increase in no., W3-5	CRVAR54, ERVAR54	If CRVAR54 < ERVAR54 then dummy=1.

Spouse

Mo. received help from outside home, W3	CSTANY	
- stopped receiving help, W3-5	CSTANY, ESTANY	If CSTANY > 0 and ESTANY < 1 then dummy=1.
No. of types of help received, W3	CSVAR54	
- decrease in no., W3-5	CSVAR54, ESVAR54	If CSVAR54 > ESVAR54 then dummy=1.
- increase in no., W3-5	CSVAR54, ESVAR54	If CSVAR54 < ESVAR54 then dummy=1.

Household

Mo. meal services received, W3	CHOMEALR	
- stopped receiving meals, W3-5	CHOMEALR, EMOMEALR	If CHOMEALR > 0 and EMOMEALR < 1 then dummy=1.
Mo. transportation service received, W3	CHOSTRAN	
Mo. attend activity center, W3	CHOCENTR	
- stopped attending, W3-5	CHOCENTR, EMOCENTR	If CHOCENTR > 0 and EMOCENTR < 1 then dummy=1.
- started attending, W3-5	CHOCENTR, EMOCENTR	If CHOCENTR < 1 and EMOCENTR > 0 then dummy=1.

APPENDIX D: TABLE 1 (continued)

DESCRIPTIVE LABELS	CORRESPONDING ANALYTIC VARIABLES	RECODING
Dwelling Configuration (multifloor units)		
Bedroom on first floor, no bath	CMSTYPE1	
Both bed and bath on first floor	CMSTYPE3	
Activity Limitations		
Respondent		
Weighted score of limitations, W3	CRSCRSUM	
- score rises, W3-5	CRSCRSUM, ERSCRSUM	If CRSCRSUM < ERSCRSUM then dummy=1.
- score falls, W3-5	CRSCRSUM, ERSCRSUM	If CRSCRSUM > ERSCRSUM then dummy=1.
Uses special equipment, W3	CRUSESEQ	
- stopped using, W3-5	CRUSESEQ, ERUSESEQ	If CRUSESEQ > ERUSESEQ then dummy=1.
- started using, W3-W5	CRUSESEQ, ERUSESEQ	If CRUSESEQ < ERUSESEQ then dummy=1.
Spouse		
Weighted score of limitations, W3	CSSCRSUM	
- score uses, W3-5	CSSCRSUM, ESSCRSUM	If CSSCRSUM < ESSCRSUM then dummy=1.
- score falls, W3-5	CSSCRSUM, ESSCRSUM	If CSSCRSUM > ESSCRSUM then dummy=1.
Uses special equipment, W3	CSUSESEQ	
- stopped using, W3-5	CSUSESEQ, ESUSESEQ	If CSUSESEQ > ESUSESEQ then dummy=1.
- started using, W3-5	CSUSESEQ, ESUSESEQ	If CSUSESEQ < ESUSESEQ then dummy=1.
Others with activity limitations present, W3	COTHRDIS	
- impaired member left, W3-5	COTHRDIS, EOTHRDIS	If COTHRDIS > EOTHRDIS then dummy=1.

Social Activity/Support

See Children weekly, W3	CSEEWKLY	
- stopped seeing children weekly, W3-5	CSEEWKLY, ESEEWKLY	If CSEEWKLY > ESEEWKLY then dummy=1.
- started seeing children weekly, W3-5	CSEEWKLY, ESEEWKLY	If CSEEWKLY < ESEEWKLY then dummy=1.
Attends church regularly, W3	CCHRCHRG	
- stopped attending regularly, W3-5	CCHRCHRG, ECHRCHRG	If CCHRCHRG > ECHRCHRG then dummy=1.
- started attending regularly, W3-5	CCHRCHRG, ECHRCHRG	If CCHRCHRG < ECHRCHRG then dummy=1.

Cost of Repairs

Average share of repairs made by: husband, spouse, other family in/out of home, W4-5	R1RSHR12-R6RSHR12	This variable equals the average value of RSHR12[b]
	R1RSHR34-R6RSHR34	This variable equals the average value of RSHR34[b]
Average cost of repairs, W2-3 ($1,000)	BAVGREP, CAVGREP	This variable equals (BAVGREP + CAVGREP)/2.

Dependent Variables[c]

Modifications Made to Unit, W4-5	DTDMOD, ETDMOD	If DTDMOD > 0 or ETDMOD > 0 then dummy=1.
Any Repair Made in Each Year, W4-5	R1ANYREP-R6ANYREP	If (R1ANYREP=1 or R2ANYREP=1 or R3ANYREP=1) and R4ANYREP=1 or R5ANYREP=1 or R6ANYREP=1) then dummy=1.
Repair Made Above Median Value[a] in Each Year, W4-5	R1TCOST-R6TCOST	If the sum of R1TCOST, R2TCOST, and R3TCOST is above the median and the sum of R4TCOST, R5TCOST, and R6TCOST is above the median then dummy=1.

189

APPENDIX D: TABLE 1 (continued)

DESCRIPTIVE LABELS	CORRESPONDING ANALYTIC VARIABLES	RECODING
Major Improvement to Unit, W4-5	RlANYMAJ-R6ANYMAJ	If any of the variables RlANYMAJ through R6ANYMAJ equal 1 then dummy=1.
No or Only Small Repairs to Unit in Each Year, W4-5	RlANYMOD-R6ANYMOD RlANYMAJ-R6ANYMAJ	If the values of RlANYMOD through R6ANYMOD and RlANYMAJ through R6ANYMAJ are all less than 1 then dummy=1.
No Repairs to Unit in Each Year, W4-5	RlANYREP-R6ANYREP	If the values for RlANYREP through R6ANYREP are all less than 1 then dummy=1.
Boarder Present, W1-5	BOARD1-BOARD5	If any of the values for BOARD1 through BOARD5 are greater than 0 then dummy=1.
Room Use Change, W3-5	CRMCHG, DRMCHG, ERMCHG	If CRMCHG=1 or DRMCHG=1 or ERMCHG=1 then dummy=1.
Dwelling Condition		
Overall structural quality, W1 - barely inhabitable - low quality	QUAL1 QUAL2	
Critical problems, W1 - foundation, walls, roof - other	CRIT1 CRIT2	
Dwelling problems present, W3	CRLEAKS, CHEATING, CTOILET, CELECT	This variable equals the sum of CRLEAKS, CHEATING, CTOILET and CELECT

Change in dwelling problems

- more, W1-3	ALEAKS, CRLEAKS,	AHEATING, CHEATING,	ATOILET, CTOILET,	AELECT CELECT	If the sum of ALEAKS, AHEATING, ATOILET, AELECT is less than the sum of CRLEAKS, CHEATING, CTOILET, CELECT, then dummy=1.
- fewer, W1-3	ALEAKS, CRLEAKS,	AHEATING, CHEATING,	ATOILET, CTOILET,	AELECT CELECT	If the sum of ALEAKS, AHEATING, ATOILET, AELECT is more than the sum of CRLEAKS, CHEATING, CTOILET, CELECT, then dummy=1.
- more, W3-5	CRLEAKS, ERLEAKS,	CHEATING, EHEATING,	CTOILET, ETOILET,	CELECT EELECT	If the sum of CLEAKS, CHEATING, CTOILET, CELECT is less than the sum of ERLEAKS, EHEATING, ETOILET, EELECT, then dummy=1.
- fewer, W3-5	CRLEAKS, ERLEAKS,	CHEATING, EHEATING,	CTOILET, ETOILET,	CELECT EELECT	If the sum of CLEAKS, CHEATING, CTOILET, CELECT is more than the sum of ERLEAKS, EHEATING, ETOILET, EELECT, then dummy=1.

Neighborhood Conditions, W1

Abandoned cars	ABCARS
House on major artery	MARTERY
Substandard houses on block	SUBSTD

Intention to Move

Likely to move, W3	CPMOVE	
- change to "likely," W1-3	ALIKEMOV, CPMOVE	If ALIKEMOV < CPMOVE then dummy=1.
- change to "not likely," W1-3	ALIKEMOV, CPMOVE	If ALIKEMOV > CPMOVE then dummy=1.
- change to "likely," W3-5	CPMOVE, EPMOVE	If CPMOVE < EPMOVE then dummy=1.
- change to "not likely," W3-5	CPMOVE, EPMOVE	If CPMOVE > EPMOVE then dummy=1.

NOTES

1. In general there was good comparability between the neighborhoods defined for the CDBG study and the Census tracts. Only for one neighborhood in Birmingham were there serious definitional problems.

2. Because of attrition over the remaining three survey waves, the attributes of the final sample will differ somewhat from those at wave 2. But we believe the wave 2 households provide a reasonable characterization of the sample.

3. In constructing the t-tests, the standard deviations used were computed for the 15 Census tracts containing the sample neighborhoods; and the difference in the mean between the sample neighborhoods and the central cities tested. It would have been more desirable to use the standard deviations for tracts in all cities (or at least a sample of all tracts). The amount of data manipulation required for this more refined test was unfortunately beyond the resources of the project.

4. The complete documentation of the imputation procedures is contained in Katsura and Struyk (1985).

5. Several individual observations had an excessive number of missing values. These observations were dropped from the sample.